# IS YOUR
# CHILD
# BIPOLAR?

# IS YOUR CHILD BIPOLAR?

*The Definitive Resource on*
*How to Identify, Treat, and Thrive*
*with a Bipolar Child*

MARY ANN McDONNELL, A.P.R.N., B.C.
AND JANET WOZNIAK, M.D.

WITH JUDY FORT BRENNEMAN

BANTAM BOOKS

IS YOUR CHILD BIPOLAR?
A Bantam Book / June 2008

Published by Bantam Dell
A Division of Random House, Inc.
New York, New York

*Book design by Carol Malcolm Russo*

Bantam Books is a registered trademark of Random House, Inc., and
the colophon is a trademark of Random House, Inc.

Library of Congress Cataloging-in-Publication Data
McDonnell, Mary Ann.
Is your child bipolar? : the definitive resource on how to identify,
treat, and thrive with a bipolar child / Mary Ann McDonnell and
Janet Wozniak with Judy Fort Brenneman.
p.   cm.
Includes bibliographical references and index.
ISBN 978-0-553-80532-1 (hardcover)
1. Manic-depressive illness in children—Popular works. I. Wozniak,
Janet. II. Brenneman, Judy Fort. III. Title.
RJ506.D4.M33 2008
618.92'895—dc22          2008010407

Printed in the United States of America
Published simultaneously in Canada

www.bantamdell.com

10 9 8 7 6 5 4 3 2 1
BVG

Although this is a work of nonfiction, we have changed names and certain identifying characteristics to protect the privacy of our patients and their families. All family stories and examples in this book are drawn from real people unless otherwise noted.

Throughout this book, we use the phrases "bipolar plus" and "plus disorders" to indicate other brain disorders that frequently occur with bipolar disorder (for example, "bipolar plus attention deficit hyperactivity disorder [ADHD]"). The formal medical term for "plus disorders" is *comorbid disorders* (for example, ADHD is a common comorbid disorder; many children who have bipolar disorder also have ADHD).

The information in this book is not intended as a substitute for consultation with healthcare professionals. Each individual's healthcare concerns should be evaluated by qualified professionals.

# Contents

*Preface*

Wednesday morning: Research and clinical staff meetings are done and it's time for the first clinic appointment of the day. The nine-year-old waiting with his parents is here for an evaluation. He and his parents want to know what's causing this young child's intense moodiness and extreme behaviors—moods and behaviors so severe that they interfere with his ability to participate in the typical activities of childhood. So disruptive that the family is in continual chaos. So alarming that they know this is something more than temperament or a rough patch.

Mental illness touches everyone. Despite the stigma often attached to mental illness, it's a rare person who doesn't know someone with—or have a relative with—a brain disorder. That's true for us, too, and one of the reasons we chose careers in child psychiatry.

When Janet's mother was in her thirties, she was diagnosed with schizophrenia. Janet's sister was an alcoholic who died at forty-six. Looking back, Janet suspects that her mother actually had a form of bipolar disorder, and that a mood disorder was hidden beneath her sister's substance abuse. Questions about the causes of psychiatric illness and what makes one person more resilient and another more susceptible led her to study psychiatry; recognizing that so many of the problems we see in adults are rooted one way or another in childhood led her to child psychiatry.

Mary Ann grew up in a large, close-knit family whose members supported and loved one another unconditionally through family struggles and tragedy. Through these life experiences, she and her family developed a better under- standing of and compassion for individuals who suffer with psychiatric disorders. They have seen the power of love and perseverance bring family members through very difficult times.

Mary Ann understands first-hand some parents' natural reactions to shrug off or ignore pathological behaviors, or to view them as "normal." She's taken care of others her whole life, including her own (now grown) children, who dealt with some of the same challenges that she did as a child. Their valuable life experiences have led two of her three children into careers in mental health, too. Empathy and insight led Mary Ann to advanced practice nursing; her first-person understanding of how challenging it is to be a child with a psychiatric disorder (or the parent of such a child) led her to child psychiatry.

Our personal experiences may have gotten us into child psychiatry, but it's the kids and their families who keep us here. Their dedication and determination to find the help their children need is awe-inspiring. Effective treatment— which includes understanding what's behind a child's difficulty as well as what to do about it—can literally change lives. That's both humbling and exciting.

By the end of today, like yesterday, like tomorrow, we will meet with many children and their families. The details of each family's story will vary, but common threads weave through all of them.

Years—eight to ten, on average—of misdiagnosis before accurate diagnosis. Treatments that made no difference or made things worse. Parents feeling helpless, hopeless, isolated, and exhausted. Kids feeling everything, but especially frustration and failure.

Some but not all of these children and teens have bipolar disorder. Many have other brain disorders in addition to or instead of bipolar. With an accurate diagnosis, appropriate treatment options, and ongoing medical care and emotional support, these children and their families can grow, learn, and thrive.

Bipolar disorder has been part of humanity for as long as there have been people. Ancient Greeks described it in both medical records and philosophical writings exploring the connections between the gods, madness, and creativity. We find descriptions of it in the histories, letters, and biographies of some of our most influential ancestors.

Sir Isaac Newton first exhibited signs of bipolar when he was a child. He graduated from college without any particular distinction, then, in the next year and a half, invented calculus, discovered why objects are different colors, and created a complete proof of the law of gravity—but he didn't publish his results until two decades later. His anger and irritability offended nearly everyone, and he endured stretches of mania and depression throughout his life. Success for Newton was defined by his fierce intellect and insatiable curiosity, not his mood disorder.

In addition to writing twenty novels, Charles Dickens founded and edited two weekly magazines, wrote thousands of letters, had a social calendar packed with friends and events in theater, the arts, and literature, was active in several charities, and still needed to walk for hours every day to work off extra energy. He also survived repeated debilitating depressions. Success for Dickens was defined by his passion for people, the arts, and social causes.

We read and hear about bipolar from people in our own day and age, too. U.S. Congressman Patrick Kennedy of Rhode Island has bipolar and continues to push for better health insurance policies for mental illnesses. Actor and author Carrie Fisher said in a 2001 interview, "You can outlast anything. It's complicated, it's a job, but it's doable.... Bipolar disorder can be a great teacher. It's a challenge, but it can set you up to be able to do almost anything else in your life."

Raising a child or teen who has bipolar is an incredibly tough job. It can be incredibly scary, too: Kids with bipolar have a greatly increased risk for substance abuse and suicide. Chaotic moods can cause severe behavior problems and disrupt every area of life.

Kids with bipolar are also some of the most remarkable kids you'll ever meet: creative and smart, resilient and strong. To help your child tap into those strengths, you need more than an accurate diagnosis and effective medical treatment. You need solid information about pediatric bipolar disorder, including what makes bipolar in kids difficult but not impossible to identify; research-based treatment, including both medical and nondrug therapies; parenting and schooling strategies; and emergency planning. Support from parents just like you who share their experiences helps, too.

That's what this book is about. We've gone beyond the plain facts and figures of what researchers and mental health specialists know about pediatric bipolar disorder. Here you'll find information about disorders that can mask or mimic bipolar as well as how we diagnose bipolar; how treatment works, with examples from real kids and their families; and ideas and strategies for school, home, and growing up. At every turn, you'll find stories from and about parents and their kids.

We'll help you make sense of bipolar so you can make sense of your child.

*Acknowledgments*

This book and the research upon which it was based would not have been possible without the education and guidance that we have received from our mentors and colleagues in the field of child psychiatry.

We are forever indebted to our mentor Dr. Joseph Biederman, chief of pediatric psychopharmacology research at Massachusetts General Hospital. Dr. Biederman inspired us with his courageous research, supported our professional endeavors, and mentored us as clinicians and researchers. He taught us to be courageous, to weather the storms of negative press that are often directed at researchers and clinicians of child psychiatry, and to not be deterred in our effort to help the very ill children whom we serve. Without his support and guidance, our level of excellence would not be what it is today.

We also thank our colleagues and the research staff at Massachusetts General Hospital and elsewhere for their support, the important work they do, and their contributions to the field of child psychiatry.

We have learned a great deal from our patients and their families. Our sincerest gratitude goes out to all of you for trusting us with your precious children and for sharing your stories and contributing to this book in an effort to help others.

## From Mary Ann McDonnell

I would like to personally thank three additional outstanding scientists and colleagues who have contributed greatly to my development as a professional.

Dr. Janet Wozniak, director of the pediatric bipolar research program at Massachusetts General Hospital and my mentor, friend, and coauthor of this book, spent endless hours sharing her expertise and contributing her research and clinical findings about pediatric bipolar disorder.

Dr. Thomas Spencer, assistant chief of pediatric psychopharmacology research at Massachusetts General Hospital, was my direct supervisor, mentor, and friend during my years at MGH. He taught me much about science and the many important aspects of research, and he also demonstrated an admirable sense of empathy, kindness, and patience in his dealings with colleagues, employees, patients, and their families. Dr. Spencer's endearing approach with patients is one that I try to model every day in my own practice.

Dr. Carol Glod, professor and research director in the School of Nursing at Northeastern University in Boston, encouraged me to pursue a career in research. She has been a consistent mentor and friend whom I have called upon many times over the years, and I thank her for her guidance and belief in my ability to succeed. She continues to play a major role in my professional development as an advisor of my PhD studies at NEU.

The unwavering love and support of my family and friends have made it possible for me to continue in my journey to help children with mental illness. I would like to especially thank my parents, Bernard and Sarah McDonnell, who have loved me unconditionally and helped me to believe that

I could accomplish whatever I set my mind to; my two brothers, Bernie and Matthew, who supported me during difficult times and celebrated with me during good times; and my three beautiful children, Christie, Jodi, and Derek, who are wonderful, loving, and always supportive of my endeavors. Their love and laughter are the driving force in my life.

## From Janet Wozniak

This book is dedicated to the hundreds of children and families who have taught me so much about pediatric bipolar disorder. You know who you are, and you know how we have been learning together about this terrible disorder, its inadequate treatments, and the often tragic outcomes. Your broken hearts fuel my endeavors to keep working.

Without Dr. Joseph Biederman I would never have learned how to really listen to the stories families were trying to tell. He is well known for his vast knowledge, clinical wisdom, and intellect, but I have to thank him most for teaching me how to think and listen. He helped free me from the previously taught notion that "children don't get bipolar disorder," so that I could truly hear what parents and children were describing. I am privileged to work with him.

I watched my mother be disabled and shamed by her psychiatric symptoms. Without that truly awful and traumatic experience, I doubt I would ever have become a psychiatrist at all. Any help I bring is a legacy to her suffering.

My own children have been the source of delight and joy in my life and have taught me what a hard job parenting is, even under the best of circumstances. They have tolerated having a mother who is divided between home and career pursuits, and I know this has not been easy for them.

My husband has supported all my endeavors 100 percent, and I want to tell him officially that he is the most important thing.

## From Judy Fort Brenneman

Thanks first and foremost to coauthors Janet Wozniak and Mary Ann McDonnell. It has been exhilarating to peek over your shoulders into the world of pediatric bipolar disorder, and it's been both a privilege and a delight to shape your extensive research and clinical experience into this book.

Thanks also to the many families who shared hard stories and hope, seasoned with a bit of humor, a dash of fury, and extra helpings of amazing determination. You are my inspiration.

When my own child was young, Dr. Tom Linnell and Dr. James Kagan helped us understand the vagaries of neurological glitches. They are a testament to all that's good in child psychology and psychiatry. Their guidance helped my child, led to my becoming a parent advocate, and put me on the path to this book, all outcomes for which I am immensely grateful.

And thanks to my family: Kyle, who taught me first-hand that there's always more than one right answer, and Ted, who keeps my world properly balanced.

## From All of Us

Thanks to our agent Jill Kneerim, of Kneerim & Williams, who guided us on the challenging path of creating a book and whose amazing memory resulted in the creative partnership between Janet, Mary Ann, and Judy. Your suggestions continue to lead us in good directions.

Thanks also to our editor Philip Rappaport and his colleagues at Bantam, who carried this book across the finish line. Your insight and expertise are greatly appreciated.

# IS YOUR CHILD BIPOLAR?

# Chapter 1

# LOST IN THE MAZE

You're exhausted.

Life with your child is chaotic. You never know what mood she'll be in from one minute to the next. A simple request might trigger a violent outburst, like the time she heaved a rock through the living room window when you asked her to set the table for supper. Something that was fine yesterday causes a major meltdown today. Last week, she tried to jump out of the car—while it was moving—when she found out that you needed to swing by the post office before picking up her friend.

You're frustrated.

Your other kids complain: *It's not fair!* You buy their sibling anything he wants. You never punish him for hitting or swearing or trashing a room. What's worse is that you know they're right. You do treat that child differently. You feel like you're always walking on eggshells just to keep the peace.

You've been looking for answers, but all you've found is confusion.

Your mother-in-law chastises you for not being strict

enough. Your child's teacher suggests ADHD. The pediatrician shrugs and reminds you that each child is different. You wonder when parenting got this hard. Maybe you remember a time when it wasn't this bad. Maybe not. Most days, you feel like you're trapped in a maze. There's no map, there are no bread crumbs to follow, and your ball of twine ran out long ago.

Parenting a child like yours is one of the toughest challenges a parent can face. Whether your son or daughter has been diagnosed with bipolar disorder or a different mood or behavior problem or behaves in ways that seem far from ordinary, this book is for you.

We can't pluck you out of the maze, but we can help you find your way through it.

Bipolar disorder is a complex illness. It doesn't look the same in everyone who has it. It often looks much different in kids than in adults. Bipolar isn't like chicken pox, where everybody's rash looks pretty much the same.

More often than not, it's "bipolar plus"—plus ADHD, depression, severe anxiety, conduct disorder, and other brain glitches.* Your child might have one, several, or many of these, which makes diagnosis and treatment challenging. Imagine waking up one morning with chicken pox, poison ivy, hay fever, and pneumonia. Where do you begin? How do you tell one from the other? Which do you treat first? Should you treat all of them? How will treating one affect the others?

Bipolar disorder has been around for as long as there have been people, but it's only been since the tail end of the twentieth century that we've started to understand what it is, how it develops, and what to do to help. Now, for the first time

---

*The formal medical term for "plus disorders" is *comorbid disorders* (for example, ADHD is a common comorbid disorder; many children who have bipolar disorder also have ADHD).

in history, solid research is joining practical experience—and the result is better diagnosis, more effective treatment, healthier kids, and happier families.

So come with us as we explore this maze. First, we'll look at the main branches: what pediatric bipolar disorder is (and isn't), why it's hard to diagnose and treat, and an overview of treatment options. Other families will chime in with their stories and experiences, too.

Think of Chapter 1 as the map that helps you get your bearings—a place to catch your breath and discover that you're not alone, and neither is your child.

## WHAT IS BIPOLAR? WHO HAS IT?

Until the early 1990s, scientists and the general public both thought bipolar disorder (also known as manic depression) was practically nonexistent in children and teens. But since 1995, research has repeatedly shown that bipolar disorder does occur in kids—and in great numbers.

According to researchers' current estimates, about 1% of all children have bipolar disorder. That means in the United States alone, more than 750,000—three-quarters of a million—children under the age of eighteen meet all the criteria for bipolar disorder. The vast majority of them—at least 80% and probably more—are undiagnosed or misdiagnosed. Evidence from adult and clinical research suggests that another 3%–4% meet the criteria for bipolar spectrum disorders, with symptoms severe enough to cause significant problems. We also know that 5% of children suffer from depression and about half of them develop bipolar disorder by the time they reach adulthood. That adds up to more than three million children in the United States with bipolar symptoms on any given day.

Obviously, they're everywhere. Why haven't you seen them?

You have. These are the kids who get labeled as "bad kids," their extreme "problem behaviors" blamed on bad parenting or violent video games. These are the kids who are diagnosed with ADHD, oppositional defiant disorder, or conduct disorder, and are treated—but the treatments either don't work or make the problem worse. Then they get new labels: "borderline personality disorder" or "incorrigible." These are the kids who get arrested for mania-induced behaviors they can't control, and the kids whose illness gets worse because treatment is nonexistent or inappropriate.

Bipolar disorder is being diagnosed in children more often than ever before, and the rate of diagnosis is increasing. Is this the "new disease of the month," a soon-to-be-forgotten fad? Is it just the latest excuse for children behaving badly?

No—absolutely not.

One of the major reasons for the increase in diagnosis is that we now recognize that the symptoms of bipolar disorder in children are much different from those of adult bipolar disorder. In addition, researchers have discovered that bipolar often exists along with other conditions that can mimic, mask, and otherwise complicate the picture. Bipolar plus one or more of these conditions is much more common in pediatric bipolar than in the adult-onset disease. We now know that bipolar disorder is the primary diagnosis in many cases that have been labeled with other names.

The actual percentage of children with bipolar disorder may be increasing, too. Studies have not yet revealed clear reasons for this.

What is completely clear is that these kids have been here all along, and they've needed help.

What's it like when your child or teen has bipolar disorder? Parents tell us—

- Every day is chaos. One minute, she's fine, the next she thinks everything is hysterically funny and she's talking a mile a minute, and a minute later she's crabby and everybody runs for cover, because we don't know if she's going to blow up or calm down.

- "Meltdown" doesn't even begin to describe it. We're talking temper tantrums that last for hours— screaming, kicking, knocking holes in the walls, the works. The doctor says a lot of kids go through a phase like this, but we've been dealing with it for a really long time and it's not getting any better.

- First, I have to deal with the stress of him exploding, then I have to listen to my husband about how I handled the situation all wrong. He thinks a lot of this is my fault.

- The teacher says he's fine at school so it must be something I'm doing wrong—but I've taken every parenting class I can find. None of them work.

- She seems fixated on anything to do with sex. The school psychologist filed a complaint with DSS, and the social worker said the behavior had to be the result of sexual abuse, but we're sure she hasn't been abused.

- We never go out anymore—we've had enough nightmares to know it isn't worth it. It's one thing when your toddler throws a tantrum at the restaurant or stands on his chair and sings a song. When you're talking about a fourteen-year-old . . .

- Our family doctor said it was ADHD, but the medication made things worse.

- It feels like her mood swings are holding us hostage. Our friends won't visit anymore, and the neighbors don't let their kids come over.

- I never know what's going to set him off. We're always walking on eggshells.

- If I knew about early-onset bipolar disorder twenty-one years ago, maybe my son would be alive today.

Bipolar disorder is a mood disorder—a mental illness that affects emotions. It's chronic and lifelong and even in adults, it can be challenging to diagnose. Adults with bipolar typically cycle through periods of low mood (depression) and high mood (mania) and may have stretches of normal mood in between. In many adults, these mood states and cycles are clear and distinct, and each emotional state can last weeks or months before cycling into the next one.

Kids with bipolar experience intense mood states, too, but most don't cycle in clear-cut patterns. Children and teens are much more likely to have mixed mood states (symptoms of both depression and mania present at the same time) and rapid cycling (switching between depression and mania very fast, many times a day, for example). This difference in how the moods change is one of the main reasons that bipolar isn't recognized in children.

The symptoms caused by moods are often different in children, too. Most of us think mania means euphoria—over-the-top silly, "flying high," lots of energy—and that depression means sad, lethargic, and joyless.

But in children, one of the most common symptoms of mania is extreme irritability, not euphoria. This manic irritability isn't the occasional grumpiness of a bad hair day. It's an irritability so extreme that it erupts in severe rages, which can include destructive, violent, or other dangerous behaviors.

Another kind of irritability shows up as a symptom of depression in children: They're whiny and exceedingly difficult to please. Parents describe their kids as snippy, snappy, grouchy, and downright nasty. Again, this is not the once-in-a-while fussiness of a tired child, the wheedling for a new toy, or disappointment that Mom said no. This is severe, intense, and disruptive.

Kids with bipolar can and do experience the other symptoms of mania and depression, but behaviors that stem from debilitating irritability are often the ones that first cause parents to seek help.

The diagnostic criteria—the symptoms you must have in order to be diagnosed—for bipolar and other mental disorders are listed in the DSM-IV (*Diagnostic and Statistical Manual of Mental Disorders*, fourth edition), the psychiatric bible relied upon throughout mental health fields to define specific illnesses and help clinicians make consistent diagnoses. Even though irritability is included as a possible symptom of bipolar, clinicians typically overlook it, especially in children; after all, irritability, like temper tantrums, is common in all kids. It can be hard for clinicians to understand that what parents are describing is not "ordinary" irritability or "typical" temper tantrums at all, but something that is severe, significant, and well beyond the ordinary. This misunderstanding about the difference between ordinary irritability and irritability from mania or depression is another reason that bipolar gets missed or misdiagnosed.

There are two other reasons that make identifying bipolar disorder in children difficult.

The first is a common misconception that bipolar symptoms only count if they happen in different settings. For bipolar, this is not true: Many kids are able to suppress their symptoms in certain situations. For example, they keep it together during school and fall apart as soon as they get home. They're not falling apart at home because there's something wrong at home; they're falling apart because they're exhausted from the effort to be "normal" at school, and home is a safe place where their friends won't see them being "crazy."

The other is the challenge of disorders that frequently occur alongside bipolar. In children, much more than in adults, it isn't just bipolar disorder causing problems; it's bipolar disorder plus one or more additional neurological glitches. For example, ADHD and bipolar can both include distractibility, impulsivity, and increased physical activity. Anxiety disorders and bipolar can both include an excessive focus on a particular task or idea. Learning disabilities and bipolar can both lead to after-school meltdowns and serious homework wars. Teachers and clinicians are more likely to notice symptoms that match illnesses and disabilities they're most familiar with and diagnose those first, not realizing that symptoms that don't quite fit are clues that the primary diagnosis is bipolar.

## HOW DO WE HELP OUR KIDS?

If you're the parent of one of these children, you know something is wrong, and you search hard for answers.

All too often, the answers you find are not helpful. Sometimes those "answers" do more harm than good. Confronted with criticism about your parenting skills and judgmental reactions from teachers, caregivers, other family members, and friends, you may become increasingly isolated, convinced that there is nowhere to turn for the information and support you and your child desperately need.

Many clinicians hesitate to diagnose and treat children who have bipolar disorder. The DSM-IV doesn't include a specific description for pediatric bipolar disorder distinct from adult-onset, and some clinicians simply refuse to believe that bipolar symptoms can appear in very young children, although there is clear evidence to support early onset, and the next edition of the DSM will likely include a section describing symptoms that are more common in children. Other clinicians believe in a "wait and see" approach, but without treatment, the illness becomes more severe. Untreated, there may be a greater chance that additional disorders will develop and treatment, when it finally begins, will be even more challenging. Some doctors do not have the knowledge to diagnose bipolar disorder in children. Their expertise lies in other areas, and they miss the hallmark symptoms.

As with any illness, timely diagnosis is crucial, but unlike strep throat or diabetes or cancer, the average time between the onset of bipolar symptoms and an accurate diagnosis is not days or weeks, but *years*—an average of *ten* years, years in which the disease worsens; the child misses critical developmental, social, and academic milestones; and the chances for a positive outcome—a healthy and productive life—continually decrease.

The good news: Parents who have been through this with their own children have formed support groups that reach out to others in neighborhoods and online. Organizations such as S.T.E.P. Up for Kids, National Alliance on Mental Illness (NAMI), and the Child and Adolescent Bipolar Foundation (CABF) provide information, education, and connections to and for parents and other professionals.

More good news: Ongoing research is leading to timely, accurate diagnosis and more effective treatment.

Treatment is driven by the type and severity of symptoms and, for most families, involves a combination of approaches. Medications help stabilize moods and manage other symptoms. Different types of psychotherapy (sometimes for your child, sometimes for you or others in your family), special educational support, and complementary or alternative healthcare can all be part of your child's treatment. Treatment—at least for now—won't cure bipolar, but it will help you and your child manage it.

Bipolar can cause behaviors that are frightening, frustrating, and infuriating. Treatment is often complex and challenging. The demands of the illness put tremendous pressure on your entire family.

And you worry: Will my child have a normal life? What will happen when he grows up? Will she find happiness and fulfillment? Go to college? Get a job? Contribute to society?

Remember that your child is not his illness. He may have bipolar; he also has unique strengths.

We can't know what gifts and talents are hidden. We can help our children discover and build on their strengths. We can nurture, guide, protect, and teach.

There are many ways to live a life, many ways to define success. Kids with bipolar have grown up to be successful in every type of job and industry, from science and engineering to performing and literary arts. The paths they traveled to get there were as varied and distinct as the individuals themselves.

Parents and other caregivers just like you helped them find their way.

| Bipolar Disorder Is NOT | Bipolar Disorder IS |
|---|---|
| Caused by bad parenting or inconsistent discipline | Caused by a combination of factors, including genetics |
| A character fault | An illness |
| Only in adults | An illness that children, including very young children, can develop |
| An excuse for bad behavior | A brain disorder: thoughts and feelings, which control behavior, come from the brain. Problems in the brain show up as problems in behavior |
| Incredibly rare in children | More common than most people realize. In the United States, there are three-quarters of a million children with full-blown bipolar, plus two to three million on the bipolar spectrum, plus one and a half million with depression who will develop bipolar by the time they're adults |
| Simple and straightforward with obvious cycles between low and high moods | Complex, chronic, and unpredictable. In children and teens, rapid cycling and mixed mood states are the rule; classic adult-style mood cycles are the exception. The number one symptom of mania is extreme irritability, not euphoria |

| Bipolar Disorder Is NOT | Bipolar Disorder IS |
| --- | --- |
| The same in all settings | Variable. Your child's symptoms might show up at home but not school, or be worse at the grocery store, or be unpredictable |
| The same in all children | A group of symptoms that includes moodiness and certain hallmark behaviors, but how the symptoms look in your child depends on many factors, including age, the severity of the bipolar illness, and whether there are other disorders present in addition to bipolar |
| "Souped up" ADHD | Sometimes mistaken for ADHD. Bipolar and ADHD do share some symptoms and many kids who have bipolar also have ADHD—but they are not the same disorder, and their treatment is different |
| Easy | One of the toughest parenting challenges out there |
| The end | Only one aspect of your child |

# Chapter 2

# DIAGNOSIS TANGLE

## IS IT REALLY—OR ONLY—BIPOLAR?

One of the first challenges you'll run into in the maze is the diagnosis tangle.

It sounds something like this.

*Susie's Teacher:* She has a hard time sitting still, and oh! what a talker! She's very high-spirited—I'm sure *you* know that!—and one of the brightest kids in class. Now, if we could only find a way to direct her energy, so she can focus and stay on task better. Perhaps it's time we had her evaluated for ADHD.

*Susie's Doctor:* It does sound like ADHD, and you say she often stays up all night to get her homework done? A little perfectionist, eh?

*Susie's Aunt:* She cried for the entire afternoon. She was convinced she'd never see home again and that something horrible was going to happen to you.

*Susie's Doctor:* Maybe an anxiety disorder . . .

*Principal at Susie's School:* This behavior is completely unacceptable. She defies every rule and twice this week, she was caught bullying other children during recess.

*Susie's Doctor:* ... or oppositional defiant disorder ...

*Susie's Girl Scout Troop Leader:* We caught her stealing. I don't think it's the first time she's done it, just the first time we've caught her. What's worse is she doesn't care. She wasn't sorry, and she laughed at me and said there wasn't anything I could do.

*Susie's Doctor:* Hmmm; it's looking more like conduct disorder ...

Each step of the way, the caring adults in Susie's life are trying to puzzle out why Susie behaves the way she does. Her behavior is a symptom that gives us clues about how her brain is working, the same way sneezing, a sore throat, and a runny nose tell us that something's bothering her nose and throat.

If you've been sneezing a lot, your throat hurts, you feel achy, and you've gone through three boxes of tissues since breakfast, there's a good chance that you've come down with a common cold. But you might have strep throat or the early stages of influenza. You go to your doctor, who checks you out thoroughly, runs a few tests, and diagnoses a cold: Go home, drink plenty of fluids, and get some rest.

Four weeks later, you don't ache as much, but you still feel miserable. You're sneezing all the time, your nose is a mess, your throat feels raw, and now your eyes are itchy and red, too. Your doctor sends you to a specialist, who identifies an allergy to the cat. You either take allergy medicine that works or give the cat to a good home, and your symptoms clear up.

Did you have a cold to begin with? Yes.

Did your symptoms go away when you recovered from the

cold? No—not until the underlying allergy was identified and treated.

It's similar with bipolar plus, though puzzling out the symptoms of thinking and feeling is harder than figuring out what's causing physical symptoms.

Mental health experts begin with the symptoms—they listen to the descriptions of your child's behavior—and identify the likely causes. Most people, including teachers, medical clinicians, and counselors as well as parents and other caring adults, are more familiar with the "plus" disorders such as ADHD and anxiety. And, until very recently, clinicians and researchers thought bipolar disorder in children was extremely rare. When a child like Susie came in for an exam, more familiar things were diagnosed, even though the symptoms didn't match completely and treatment couldn't solve the whole problem.

Effective treatment depends on accurate diagnosis. Susie might have ADHD, anxiety disorder, and conduct or oppositional defiant disorder, which of course need to be addressed, but if Susie's bipolar disorder isn't treated first, treatment for the other problems won't be effective.

Sorting out what is going on is tricky. The behaviors and symptoms caused by the plus disorder can make it hard to tell what is causing a particular problem. One disorder can mimic or hide another. Is your child unable to sit still in school because of ADHD, mania, both, or something else? The right answer for yesterday's antics may be the wrong one for today's. Treatment for one condition may aggravate symptoms in another. Treatment for the wrong disorder, perhaps because of an incorrect diagnosis, can have disastrous results.

Sometimes, it's clear that your child or teen has bipolar disorder. More often, you'll have to untangle a snarled heap of symptoms and possible causes to figure out if it's bipolar, bipolar plus, or another condition entirely.

Let's begin with the symptoms: behaviors that raise red flags.

Behaviors are clues; we observe them to figure out what's going on. As a parent, you've been doing that from the very beginning. When your baby gurgled and cooed, you knew he was happy and content. When he fussed or cried, you suspected that he was hungry, needed a diaper change, or wanted to be cuddled. As he grew, you got better at figuring out the clues: This cry meant he was hungry, that shriek meant he'd thrown Bobo the Bear out of his crib again. General fussiness meant time for a nap, but fussiness with lots of ear rubbing probably meant an ear infection.

As kids grow, they pass through developmental stages. We expect certain behaviors and abilities at certain ages. For example, no one would be surprised if your toddler started crying when you dropped her off at the day care she'd gone to without difficulty every day since she was a baby, because separation anxiety is normal in toddlers. But it will raise some eyebrows if your fifteen-year-old refuses to let you out of her sight and cries nonstop when you try to take her to school.

For the toddler, separation anxiety is developmentally appropriate; it's part of normal development. It shows up as early as eighteen months and usually drops away by the third birthday. Separation anxiety in a teenager is not developmentally appropriate; it tells us something is out of kilter.

Behavior that shows up at an inappropriate developmental stage is an important clue, but we need two other clues from behavior before trying to diagnose what's going on.

The first is severity: Does your toddler settle in quickly or does she keep crying, no matter how skillfully the preschool teacher tries to redirect her attention? Does she cry for five minutes? ten? until she collapses from exhaustion?

The second is frequency: How often does the behavior occur? Does your teenaged daughter cry and refuse to go to school every day? Once in a blue moon? Four times last week when she broke up with her boyfriend?

Every child has moments when they worry, throw tantrums, get distracted, challenge their parents, are impulsive, and get into mischief (usually not all at the same time!). It's true that some kids are more willful or impulsive than others. Some children seem to be born worriers and others love risk and adventure. But when a behavior or group of behaviors is frequent and severe enough to get in the way of ordinary day-to-day life, there's more going on than temperament.

We'll talk about the specific symptoms of bipolar disorder in Chapter 3, but before we get there, let's look at the disorders that often show up alongside bipolar: the "plus" of bipolar plus. These are the disorders you and your child's teachers and clinician may already be familiar with. They're the disorders that often get blamed for causing bipolar symptoms, and they're the ones that can trip up effective treatment.

## ATTENTION DEFICIT HYPERACTIVITY DISORDER

ADHD (or ADD, AD/HD) is the most common plus condition we see.

About 5% of the general population—one child out of twenty—has ADHD. The rate is much higher among kids who have bipolar. In those whose bipolar disorder began in adolescence, 50%—ten out of twenty—have ADHD. In those who develop bipolar before the age of twelve, over 90%—eighteen out of twenty—have ADHD. Looking at this another way, 1% (one out of a hundred) of the general population has bipolar disorder, but among the population of kids who have ADHD, 20% (one out of five) have bipolar disorder.

Many of the children who come to us for evaluation have at some time been misdiagnosed either as having ADHD when in fact they have bipolar, or they have both ADHD and bipolar but only the ADHD was identified. This is a serious problem because the drugs used to treat ADHD can make the bipolar symptoms worse. When a child has both disorders, the bipolar symptoms must be stabilized first, before adding ADHD medications.

ADHD's symptoms fall into three categories: inattention, hyperactivity, and impulsivity. The DSM-IV divides ADHD into three subtypes, based on the symptoms your child has.

• *Inattentive subtype, without hyperactivity or impulsivity.* Kids with the inattentive subtype are easily distracted. They space out, wander off on field trips, and miss directions. They may miss social cues. They might not do well in school because they make careless mistakes and forget to turn in their homework, even when they're reminded. They generally aren't disruptive and their difficulties are often minimized—they're called dreamers, absentminded professors, and scatterbrains.

• *Hyperactive/impulsive subtype.* Kids with this subtype can't sit still (their teachers call them jack-in-the-boxes because they pop out of their chairs so often). They talk nonstop, can't play quietly, act impulsively without thinking about consequences and then regret what they've said or done. They're fidgety (teens may be able to sit still when they have to, but they may feel extremely restless) and have a hard time waiting their turn. They're liable to blurt out their thoughts the moment they think them.

• *Combined subtype.* Kids with this subtype have both inattentive and hyperactive/impulsive symptoms.

To be diagnosed with ADHD, your child has to have enough of the symptoms, and the symptoms must be inappropriate for the developmental level (an older child should be able to wait his turn, a younger child is still learning how to wait); frequent and severe enough to be disruptive; and not caused by something else (another mental disorder, for example).

The combined subtype is the most common; 50%–75% of

all people with ADHD have this subtype. It's also the subtype most frequently confused with bipolar disorder.

Bipolar and the combined subtype of ADHD have three symptoms that overlap or look very similar: The pressured speech of mania can be mistaken for the excessive talking of ADHD; the increased physical activity and poor judgment that are part of bipolar can look like ADHD's hyperactivity and impulsivity; and distractibility is common in both disorders.

There are critical differences between ADHD and bipolar disorder, which an experienced clinician can usually identify in a careful evaluation.

ADHD is not a mood disorder; it's a neurological glitch that affects impulse control and the ability to direct and focus attention. Kids with ADHD don't have severe and frequent mood changes. The symptoms of ADHD don't begin suddenly, and they don't fluctuate the way bipolar symptoms do. When a child with ADHD throws a temper tantrum, it's usually triggered by the stress of needing to be still, pay attention, or cope with too much stimulation. The tantrums can be loud and disruptive, but they're usually over quickly. Tantrums in kids with bipolar are most often triggered by limit setting and conflict with authority, and they can last literally for hours. (And, as we'll discuss in Chapter 3, these episodes aren't normal, developmentally appropriate temper tantrums, but severe outbursts or *rage storms*.)

If your child has bipolar plus ADHD, regardless of which subtype, we begin by treating the bipolar disorder. Sometimes, the ADHD symptoms resolve as your child's moods stabilize. In other cases, your child may still experience some ADHD challenges. Those ADHD symptoms might be minor and respond well to nonmedical support or significant enough that we'll treat it with medication that works with his bipolar treatment, instead of against it.

For additional descriptions of ADHD symptoms, see Appendix B.

### Trevor: ADHD, definitely with H!

"Exuberant" is the first word that comes to mind when watching Trevor. Within ten minutes, he's dumped all the LEGO bricks on the floor and begun and abandoned half a dozen structures. He spies a stack of paper and colored pencils and stretches out on the floor to draw. After changing his mind several times about which pencil to use, he tosses off a series of fast sketches, handing each one to his mom as he finishes. He jumps up from the floor, knocking over the canister of pencils. He dumps the pencils back into the canister and shoves the canister out of the way, then starts digging through the LEGO pile again.

Trevor's generally upbeat, cheerful, and talkative—very talkative. He interrupts the conversation and rattles on about things that may not have anything to do with the topic at hand. His monologues wander so much that it's hard to follow what he's saying or figure out what point he's trying to make. When he was younger, he had a hard time controlling his temper, especially in noisy or crowded places.

Trevor's small for his age, so watching his antics, it's easy to forget that he's not a rambunctious seven-year-old; he's almost thirteen.

Trevor is impulsive and hyperactive at school—so much so that he's behind where he should be academically—and at home, too. He's enthusiastic and comes up with great ideas, but unfinished projects (including homework and chores) follow him everywhere.

### Elyssa: ADHD, inattentive type

"A social butterfly," the teachers tell Elyssa's parents. "Plenty of friends, and she's never a problem"—which is more a comparison to Elyssa's older brother, who is not a social butterfly and is in trouble all the time. She gets caught daydreaming in class often enough that her teachers remark on it. She's not rude or deliberately ignoring the teacher; she's just "spacey." Still, everyone is relieved that Elyssa is sweet and charming and is passing all her classes.

Elyssa's parents are a little concerned because although she's passing, Elyssa's grades are only so-so. She seems so much brighter than that. At parent-teacher night, all of Elyssa's teachers tell them the same thing. Ninth grade can be a challenging transition. If Elyssa were more organized, it might help; she's always losing track of her assignments and rarely turns in her homework. She'd do better on her tests if she'd be more careful. And she really needs to learn to keep an eye on the clock— she'd been tardy to several classes, especially math, which is right after lunch.

Because Elyssa's easy-going and well behaved, there's a real risk that her ADHD will go undiagnosed. Her teachers are describing typical symptoms of inattentive ADHD: disorganized, losing track of things, losing track of time, careless mistakes—symptoms her parents have noticed at home, too, in different form, such as losing library books, the last-minute scramble to collect her things for school, and forgetting chores or getting sidetracked halfway through and not finishing. She will need more than organizational strategies and time management to reach her potential.

## ANXIETY DISORDERS

Another common plus disorder is anxiety. Roughly half of children and teens with bipolar also have two or more anxiety disorders. Sometimes there's something specific that triggers the onset of an anxiety disorder or certain stresses that make it worse, but there doesn't have to be.

Anxiety means fears or worries that are so intense they cause problems in your child's day-to-day life. She might have trouble falling asleep or concentrating at school because she's worrying so much. She might avoid places or situations that she's afraid of—or is worried that she'll be afraid of. She might be clingy or complain about tummy aches or other physical symptoms. Whatever form her anxiety takes, it is frequent enough and severe enough to interfere with normal activities.

There are nine types of anxiety disorders, and it isn't unusual to have more than one type. The types are divided in part by what the child's worry or fear is focused on—fear of being separated from his parents is a different category than fear of spiders, for example—but beyond these different focuses, we don't know how and why anxiety disorders appear in such variety. We do know that a panic attack may contribute to a specific phobia or to agoraphobia. We know symptoms wax and wane and that the two most disabling anxiety disorders in children and teens are obsessive-compulsive disorder and panic disorder. We suspect that some types of anxiety disorders may shift into other types as the child grows up. We also know—as with other plus disorders—that children with anxiety disorders who aren't treated are at greater risk for poor school performance, substance abuse, and delays in social skills development.

The nine types of anxiety disorders are specific phobias, panic disorder, agoraphobia, separation anxiety, social anxiety, avoidant disorder, post-traumatic stress disorder, obsessive-compulsive disorder, and overanxious disorder (in adolescents and adults, this last one is called *generalized anxiety disorder*).

## SPECIFIC PHOBIAS

A phobia is an intense, irrational fear of a specific thing. Common phobias include fear of a particular kind of animal (spiders, for example), certain situations (flying), or something abstract, such as the number thirteen.

Many kids go through phases where they're afraid of something; dogs, storms, and the dark are all common childhood fears. But if your child's fear has lasted for six months or more and is severe enough to disrupt his normal activities, it's a phobia.

If you, an adult, have ophidiophobia—fear of snakes—you can probably tell your friends that you won't go hiking with them because you're too afraid of encountering a snake. You know your fear is out of proportion to the risk involved (though knowing that doesn't mean you'll go on the hike) and you're aware that you avoid certain activities and situations because of the fear.

Unlike adults, kids don't always understand that the intensity of their fear doesn't match the danger of the object or situation. They may not be able to tell you that they're afraid; they may not recognize or be able to describe their fear. It shows up in their behavior: If they can, they'll avoid what they fear. You may not know that the reason your son refuses to play outside is because he's afraid there might be snakes. What you know is that he used to enjoy being outside but now he won't go out, even if he wants to.

If a child can't avoid the scary situation, he'll do his best to endure it, and his anxiety and fear will show up in behavior. He'll cry, cling, throw a tantrum, or complain of headaches and tummy aches.

## PANIC DISORDER

Panic disorder is an especially severe type of anxiety. It involves distinct episodes called *panic attacks*. During a panic attack, you experience specific physical symptoms and intense feelings of doom—you literally feel like you're going to die. The physical symptoms are the same ones you get when your body goes into "fight-or-flight"—which makes sense, because your brain is convinced that something terrible is about to befall you. What doesn't make sense is why your brain is convinced of this.

Panic is a legitimate reaction to significant and immediate danger. If you are being attacked by a lion, your brain sends out the signals that make you fight harder, run faster, scream louder—to do whatever it takes to get to safety.

Panic attacks are the same reaction, except there isn't a danger; there is no lion.

Panic attacks can result in specific phobias. Since the panic is spontaneous and not triggered by a known danger, your brain might associate the panic with whatever is nearby. If you happened to be on an escalator when the attack hit, you might develop a phobia about escalators.

Whether your panic reaction connects itself to something else or stays free-floating, it feels so awful that you become afraid of having another attack. You begin to avoid places that remind you of where you've had attacks. You avoid places and situations you can't leave quickly and easily. A child who refuses to go to school might not be fearful or anxious about school itself, but might be afraid of having a panic attack in the classroom, convinced that there's no way to escape if she has an attack. This kind of avoidance can develop into full-fledged agoraphobia, which is another type of anxiety disorder.

## AGORAPHOBIA

Contrary to popular belief, agoraphobia isn't simply a fear of being in an open space. It's the fear of being in a place or situation you can't escape from. It often develops alongside panic disorder: If you're afraid of having a panic attack, you're going to avoid places where escape is difficult (remember, panic attacks push your fight-or-flight reaction). Kids and adults with agoraphobia may be anxious or afraid of crowds, small spaces (claustrophobia is actually a type of agoraphobia), being in the house or a room alone, or leaving the house or other familiar setting. People with severe agoraphobia may become housebound—so afraid that they are unable to leave.

## SEPARATION ANXIETY

Many kids go through a phase where they don't want to let their parents out of sight. They fuss if Mom steps into the kitchen and they can't follow. They cry when dropped off at Grandma's. They balk (sometimes loudly) at going to preschool. By the time they're four, most of them have outgrown their separation anxiety.

Some kids don't outgrow it, and others begin to experience it again when they're older. The anxiety is centered specifically around separation from loved ones, usually a parent or other significant caregiver.

Kids with this type of anxiety disorder feel miserable when they're not in direct contact with their parent. At school or camp (assuming you can get them to go at all), they are extremely homesick. They may worry nonstop that something terrible will happen to their parents while they're apart. When they are in contact with Mom or Dad, they're often in literal contact, clinging, following closely no matter where Mom or Dad goes, insisting that Mom or Dad stay with them at bedtime.

## SOCIAL ANXIETY

Kids with social anxiety aren't just shy. They're terrified of social and performance situations. They want to be sociable, to have friends and join in social activities, but they fear and try to avoid unstructured peer activities (playing with others at recess, going to a party), speaking up in class, starting conversations, inviting friends to get together, and anything to do with performing in front of others. Because they avoid as much of these normal interactions as possible, they miss out—on friendship, school, and developing the skills to build and maintain relationships.

## AVOIDANT DISORDER

Avoidant disorder in kids looks a lot like social anxiety disorder. Current thinking is that in children and teens, avoidance disorder is a variation on social anxiety disorder, not a separate category of anxiety as it is for adults.

Children and teens with avoidant disorder don't adjust easily to new people or new situations. They're afraid of criticism, disapproval, and rejection. They're reluctant to try anything new because they believe they'll be shamed or ridiculed. Their fears are even greater when the situations involve people they don't know. Sometimes avoidant disorder may be mistaken for separation anxiety because the behavior of avoiding unfamiliar people and places can look the same as the behavior of refusing to separate from the most familiar people in the child's life, his parents.

## POST-TRAUMATIC STRESS DISORDER

Post-traumatic stress disorder (PTSD) is an anxiety disorder related to a specific incident. Usually, the incident was terrifying and involved physical harm or the threat of physical harm. A child with PTSD might have directly experienced the harm or threat or might have witnessed a harmful event that happened to someone else. Kids who have suffered physical or sexual abuse, lived through an earthquake, hurricane, or war, or who have witnessed these things may develop PTSD.

Not everyone who experiences a traumatic event develops PTSD; some may develop depression or a different anxiety disorder. For those who do develop PTSD, symptoms range from relatively mild to incapacitating. Kids with PTSD may experience many of the symptoms seen in the other anxiety disorders (crying, clinging, avoiding situations, tantrums), but they also have symptoms specific for PTSD, related to the trauma. Kids with PTSD may "relive" the event over and over through strong memories, flashbacks, nightmares, and intrusive thoughts (they can't stop thinking about the event). They may have trouble sleeping, startle easily, and be irritable. They might become more aggressive or violent as they mentally re-experience the trauma. They may feel emotionally numb and lose interest in things they used to enjoy.

## OBSESSIVE-COMPULSIVE DISORDER

As its name implies, obsessive-compulsive disorder (OCD) has two parts:

Obsessive thoughts—thoughts that are persistent and
    upsetting, and
Compulsive behavior—ritual-like behaviors done
    over and over in an attempt to alleviate the
    anxiety caused by the obsessive thought.

Sometimes there's a clear link between the obsessive thought and the compulsive behavior. For example, if your son is obsessed with germs, he might wash his hands over and over.

Other compulsive behaviors don't have an obvious link. Your daughter might have to touch five things in her room before she leaves, and if she doesn't touch them in the right way and the proper sequence, she has to start over. If you ask her why, she may not have a reason, rational or otherwise. If you insist that she leave her room before she's finished, her anxiety may be so severe that she can't leave the room, and if you carry her out, she may cry, throw a tantrum, or behave in other ways that let you know she's afraid.

Almost anything can become an obsessive thought or compulsive behavior, but the more common ones include obsessions with germs or disease, intruders, harming others, sex, and thoughts that are prohibited by the person's religious beliefs. Common compulsions (or rituals) include hand-washing, locking and relocking doors and windows, repeatedly checking things, touching things (especially in a particular sequence), and counting (for example, counting the number of steps it takes to reach the mailbox). Sometimes kids and adults with OCD need to have things "evened up"; it bothers them when things aren't in a particular order or aren't symmetrical. At the same time, they may hoard things they don't need and have a hard time throwing things away. The resulting clutter can look like the disorganized mess of a child who has ADHD, but the reaction of the child when you try to help clean (or demand that they do it themselves) will be much different.

## OVERANXIOUS DISORDER

Kids who have overanxious disorder worry about all kinds of things, from grades and how well they're doing in sports to how bad the next earthquake will be. These kids tend to be very hard on themselves. They may redo a task again and again, trying to be perfect. They can't control their extreme worry and they may need constant reassurance. Their anxiety makes them restless, irritable, and physically tense. They may have trouble concentrating or sleeping because they are worrying so much, and being tired makes it harder for them to concentrate, which makes them worry more. They may complain about headaches, tummy aches, and other physical symptoms that don't appear to have a physical cause.

### Owen: Panic Disorder and Specific Phobias

Owen is afraid of clouds. Not storm clouds that menace and rumble with thunder, not the solid gray masses that turn winter days to twilight long before sunset, but big, white, puffy clouds, the kind that float serenely in lazy summer skies, the ones other kids gaze at in wonder and delight, imagining distant magical kingdoms.

Owen's mom didn't know about the clouds. What she did know was that Owen was afraid of many things, none of which made sense. He was afraid to go outside and when she insisted, he'd hang on to her the whole time—which might have been fine when he was a toddler, but he was almost five now. He was afraid of cars, though she could usually get him into their minivan, provided it was parked in the garage and he could sit in the center of the middle seat. He was afraid of the toy box in the family room but not the one in his bedroom.

She didn't think he was afraid of the dark, but he wouldn't fall asleep unless the curtains were drawn completely and his dad was in the room. If he woke during the night and Dad wasn't there, he'd cry until his dad came back. More than once, Dad has fallen asleep on the beanbag chair next to Owen's bed; everybody gets more sleep that way.

What worries Owen's parents most is that the list of things he's afraid of is getting longer, and even when he's not obviously scared, he seems anxious and worried. "Mommy's little huggy-bear," his mom calls him when her friends comment on how much reassurance he needs—but lately, to herself, she's been thinking, "Mommy's little leech-boy."

At first, Owen's doctor thought Owen was just a little slow in outgrowing separation anxiety, but the intensity of Owen's anxiety plus the fact that he was anxious so much of the time suggested something more serious. Maybe overanxious disorder, since he was afraid of so many things? That didn't seem to fit Owen exactly; yes, he was often anxious and fearful, but in some situations, he was just fine. And most of his fears seemed so specific.

Gradually, Owen, his parents, and the doctor sorted out what was going on: Owen was having panic attacks, and had probably been having them from the time he was very young. The fears he struggled with now were a direct result of panic disorder. Along the way, they also figured out that Owen wasn't afraid of going outside—he was afraid of clouds, and had been for as long as he could remember. There's no way to know for sure when he had his first panic attack, but they suspect it was outside on a sunny day, when big fluffy clouds happened to be floating overhead.

### Rhea: OCD

Rhea's room is a wreck. There's enough clutter to fill three rooms. Blankets and stuffed animals overflow the bed. The bookshelves are crammed and more books and papers are piled in haphazard stacks on the floor, in front of the dresser, and under the window. Her dresser and closet are jam-packed with clothes, some that fit but most, like the stuffed animals, she outgrew long ago. Rhea refuses to throw out any of her "favorites," clothes or toys, though last summer she did agree to let her mom store some things in a box that now rests on the rafters in the garage, where she can see it every morning. The box has a label on each side with her name in big red letters.

The top of Rhea's dresser is cluttered, too, but in an entirely different way. There's a sheet of plywood on top of the dresser, and on top of that, there's a piece of white cotton the same size as the plywood. On top of that is an entire village of Little People toys. It's the medieval setting and has everything a storybook village should have, from castles with towers to dragons, fair maids, and knights on horseback, complete with small plastic lances.

Rhea knows where every character, building, animal, and prop is in the village. She checks regularly to make sure nothing's been moved, sometimes picking up a piece and setting it back down to make sure it is in exactly the right place. Sometimes she's still not sure, so she picks it up and replaces it, making minute adjustments many times before she's satisfied. When asked, she says she can tell the piece is in the right place because it feels right.

That's why she divides raspberries into groups of four—if there's five in the bowl, it doesn't feel right—and why she used to count Cheerios, also in multiples of four (she'll measure out one-fourth of a cup four times now instead of counting individual pieces of cereal).

Rhea's family might think of these things as quirks, small eccentricities in their bright, creative little girl—but sometimes Rhea is up way past bedtime, checking and rechecking the village on the dresser. She misses the school bus at least once a week because she has to run back inside just one more time to make sure nothing's moved. Her insistence on counting pieces of food has delayed supper so often that her mom tries to fix foods that can't be divided, like oatmeal or chili (without beans; Rhea counts the beans). And when her parents insist that she "just eat your supper, please," Rhea cries, refuses, or throws a tantrum.

### Shelly: OCD

Shelly is a straight-A student in the gifted and talented program at her elementary school. She's officially a fourth-grader, but she's doing junior-high level work. She loves her school, her teachers, her classes, her friends—which is why everyone was surprised when she started arriving late to school almost every day.

School was only five blocks from home, and Shelly had walked it with her sisters almost every day since kindergarten. She was still walking but often, they'd get partway there and she'd stop, turn around, and run back home, saying she'd forgotten something. The first few times, her sisters waited for her, but sometimes Shelly had to go back more than once, so they gave up and went to school without her.

Shelly's mom didn't know she'd come home again, because Shelly didn't come inside the house. The first Mom heard about it was when a teacher called. School had started over an hour ago and Shelly wasn't there. Her sisters said she'd gone back home; was everything okay?

Shelly's mom found her halfway between school and home, exhausted and crying.

At home, the story began to come out. Shelly had to count her steps to school. A math project? No, she just had to count. And if she lost count, she had to go home and start over. Counting began from the first step of the porch and ended when she entered the school building. When her mom asked her what would happen if she didn't count, Shelly said, "It feels like I'll die."

It turned out that Shelly had been counting lots of things for a long time. She didn't remember when it started, only that she thought about it a lot. She didn't know that other people didn't count and think about counting all the time; she assumed what she was experiencing was normal and that she just wasn't handling it as well as everybody else was. And counting steps to school was harder than anything else she'd been counting. The day the school called, she'd made the trip partway to school and back eight times by the time her mom found her.

## PERVASIVE DEVELOPMENTAL DISORDER (PDD) AND AUTISTIC SPECTRUM DISORDER (ASD)

Pervasive developmental disorder (PDD), which includes autism and Asperger's syndrome, is a category of disorders characterized by problems in socialization and communication. Autistic spectrum disorder (ASD) is beginning to replace the term PDD because it's a more accurate description. Children (and adults) with these disorders vary widely in severity of symptoms, intelligence, behaviors, and degree of disability. Some kids are profoundly affected and have serious difficulties. Others are "high-functioning" and, with the right supports, make their way in life successfully. A child who falls somewhere on the autistic spectrum but whose symptoms don't meet the DSM-IV criteria for autism or Asperger's syndrome might be diagnosed with PDD-NOS: pervasive developmental disorder, not otherwise specified. Asperger's syndrome and PDD-NOS are more common than autism, and any of them can be a plus disorder.

ASD is a developmental disorder, not a mental illness or emotional disorder. Kids with ASD have problems with communication. They don't pick up on social cues and nonverbal clues such as eye contact, facial expressions, and body language that are part of social interactions. They have a hard time making and keeping friends because social interactions don't make sense to them.

Children with autism usually have speech delays and, if their speech is adequate, their language may be unusual, with repeated phrases or statements that seem unrelated to the situation. Speech and language development in children who have Asperger's usually isn't delayed, but it may be unusual, with odd inflections, accents, or a stilted tone. Kids with Asperger's (whether their speaking voice sounds normal or not) may launch unbidden into enthusiastic outpourings about their favorite topic—whether or not the listener is interested. Engaging in actual conversation, where each person takes turns and the topic can change, is often a major challenge.

These kids may also flap their hands, spin, rock, or do other repetitive movements or behaviors, especially when they're upset or feeling distressed. Some have a strong need for ritual and routine. At first glance, many of these behaviors might be mistaken for symptoms of other plus disorders. The Asperger's combination of nonstop talking and missing social cues can look like the ADHD chatterbox or the talkativeness of mania in bipolar. But the child with ADHD interrupts impulsively and the things she talks about are liable to be all over the map, instead of focused on the details of a single topic. The speech mannerisms of a child with Asperger's will range from ordinary to stilted; you won't hear the rapid-fire pressured speech common in mania.

Temper tantrums that erupt are usually the result of sensory overload or disrupted rituals and routines, similar to ADHD and OCD, but can also be from the frustration of trying to figure out the social and emotional world that doesn't make sense to most of these kids.

A significant minority of kids with ASD have irritability and aggressive behavior, big reactions to little triggers, distractibility, and physical agitation (needing to move), all symptoms common in bipolar disorder. Inflexible thinking can also be part of both. ADHD is a common plus disorder in each of them, too.

In children who have only ASD, symptoms are constant in their lives. In children who have only bipolar disorder, there isn't a consistent pattern. For example, a child with ASD may insist on a routine every day, no matter what; breaking the routine results in a huge tantrum or other extreme behavior. A child with bipolar might be that rigid and inflexible during a manic episode, but when her mood is stable, her ability to cope is similar to that of children who don't have brain disorders. A child with both has a much more compromised course than a child who has only one or the other.

### Jason: Autism
Jason was diagnosed with autism when he was four. He has lots of behaviors common in kids who have autism—rocking, spinning, tapping, hand-flapping—especially when he is upset or overwhelmed. When he was younger, he threw horrible temper tantrums that included banging his head on the floor. He still throws occasional tantrums, usually when he's feeling completely overloaded. Although Jason can talk, his speech is limited to short repeated phrases of things he's heard in movies or on TV.

He began attending public school when he was five, first entirely in a special ed program designed for kids with similar disabilities. Now, as a seven-year-old, he spends part of each day in the mainstream classroom, too, with a paraprofessional assigned to work with him as an in-class aide.

Things in the mainstream class started out well, but about halfway through the semester, Jason's behavior before, during, and after mainstream started to deteriorate. It hadn't escalated to temper tantrums, but there was plenty of hand-flapping and rocking. Clearly, something was wrong, but what?

At the end of an especially trying week, the mainstream teacher called the special ed teacher to come collect Jason. They'd just watched the movie *Pinocchio* as a special treat—in fact, she'd picked the movie because she knew Jason loved it, and she thought it might cheer him up. Instead, he got more agitated.

On the way back to the special ed classroom, Jason kept repeating a line from the movie: "I want to be a real boy. I want to be a real boy." Most days, his teacher wouldn't have given such repetition a second thought—Jason repeated lines from cartoons, commercials, and movies all the time, and they never seemed to mean anything. This time, she thought about behavior as communication; was there more to this today than calming repetition?

She did a little investigating and discovered that Jason's first in-class aide had moved to another school about the same time Jason started having problems. The new paraprofessional was well trained and enthusiastic, but she felt that since she was Jason's aide, she should stay right next to him for the entire class time. The previous aide had given Jason plenty of help, but she moved back and forth among the other students, lending a hand when they needed, coming back to Jason when he needed her. To Jason, the first in-class aide treated him like all the other kids—he was a "real boy" just like they were. He didn't want—and didn't really need—the aide by his side every minute. The new aide agreed to try roaming among all the students, and Jason settled back into the classroom.

### Scott: Asperger's Syndrome

Scott is the neighborhood computer geek. He eats, breathes, and sleeps computers; it's his number one passion. Actually, it's his *only* passion. Family members have learned to tolerate his long-winded explanations of programs and networks and arcane commands—after all, he keeps the home system up and running, not to mention the computers of half the relatives. Listening to Scott talk about computers is like trying to sip from a firehose; there is no way to get just a little information. You get everything, no matter how minute or relevant the detail, and you can't shift the topic, let alone change it. Scott doesn't mind if you interrupt him, but he'll go right back to where he was in the computer conversation, no matter that your eyes have glazed over.

## OPPOSITIONAL DEFIANT DISORDER

Kids who have a pattern of negative, hostile, and defiant behaviors for at least six months may have oppositional defiant disorder (ODD).

Children and teens with ODD often lose their tempers. They argue with adults and challenge authority at every turn. They're touchy, irritable, and easily annoyed. Some are angry and resentful, or spiteful and vindictive (or all of the above). When they make mistakes or misbehave, it's always someone else's fault.

Sort of sounds like your typical rebellious teen, doesn't it?

The difference is that kids with ODD don't do this once in a while to test their wings; they do this frequently and severely enough that it gets in the way of school, friendships, family relationships, work, and other activities.

ODD is diagnosed only if the behaviors are not part of a psychotic or mood disorder—which is especially important, because new research suggests ODD, like its more serious cousin conduct disorder (described in the next section), is often tightly linked to pediatric bipolar disorder; it is the second most common plus disorder.

In fact, ODD seldom occurs all on its own, and there seem to be different forms of it. Some forms are linked to ADHD, some to depression, others to conduct disorder or sociopathy, and still others to pediatric bipolar disorder. Additional plus disorders make the picture even more complicated. For example, the impulsivity and hyperactivity of ADHD—the most common plus disorder—can fuel the symptoms of ODD. Identifying the conditions that are present along with ODD can aid in treatment.

Until recently, treatment for ODD focused on structured behavioral approaches, for example, contracts that clearly spelled out the rules and consequences and were consistently applied by everyone working with the child. These methods are still appropriate and effective for many children, but treating underlying problems that do respond well to medication—

bipolar and ADHD being top examples—often helps the ODD, too. A new technique, collaborative problem solving (CPS), offers another approach to treating ODD that doesn't rely on behavioral rewards and consequences. (For more on CPS, see Chapter 8.)

## CONDUCT DISORDER

Conduct disorder (CD) has all the challenges of ODD and adds in mean, cruel, or dishonest behavior. CD is not just children being bad; it is the precursor to criminality. To be diagnosed with CD, the behavior must include violating basic rights of others or breaking major rules and values of society. These behaviors are divided into four groups:

- Aggression to people and animals, including bullying, using a weapon to cause harm, physical cruelty to people and animals, and sexual assault

- Destruction of property by fire or other means

- Deceitfulness or theft, including conning someone, shoplifting, and forgery

- Serious violations of rules, including running away, staying out all night, and skipping school

The behaviors of conduct disorder are severe and frequent; playing hooky one time isn't conduct disorder, nor is the occasional bad choice kids make. Boys with CD are more likely to fight, steal, and destroy property. Girls are more likely to lie, run away, and be involved in severe social acting out, including prostitution.

Kids with conduct disorder often seem to misinterpret the intentions of other people, but unlike kids with ASD (who misunderstand social cues in a variety of ways), they believe others are threatening or criticizing them. They respond with aggressive behavior and, other than anger or self-righteousness, show little emotion or remorse. Kids with ADHD sometimes react aggressively, too, but afterward, when they've calmed down, they are usually sad and sorry for what they've done.

Kids with CD are often reckless, but their disregard for normal safety issues isn't the same as the impulsive or thrill-seeking behavior we see in ADHD. The reckless behavior of CD is similar to behaviors we see in some kids who have bipolar.

Emerging research suggests that some cases of ODD and CD are fueled by bipolar disorder, ADHD, or depression (or a combination). There is a big overlap between ODD and CD, and an even bigger overlap between these and bipolar disorder—enough so that we suspect bipolar plus ODD, CD, or both may be a distinct bipolar subtype.

Conduct disorder, like ODD, has been a tough treatment challenge. Structured behavioral approaches, including contracts that clearly define actions, expectations, and consequences, sometimes help.

Because there aren't specific medical treatments for ODD and CD, clinicians look for underlying problems, including bipolar and ADHD, that may be causing or aggravating the ODD and CD. Treating the underlying disorder should ease or eliminate the ODD and CD.

When a child who is irritable, grandiose, and impulsive begins to lie, steal, bully, or vandalize, we want to know if this is a case where the child is a criminal in the making, a child with out-of-control mania, or both. Treating the mania may derail the budding "criminal career"—important for both the individual child and society as a whole.

## LEARNING DISABILITIES

Learning disabilities (LDs; sometimes called *learning differences*) encompass a broad group of disorders that stem from problems in understanding or using spoken or written language. Kids with LDs often have average or above-average intelligence, but their disability trips them up; they aren't able to do as well as we expect them to. This mismatch between the child's potential and her performance is often one of the first clues suggesting LD.

LDs are often language processing disorders, which means there's a glitch somewhere in how the brain receives, interprets, and responds to spoken or written language. Dyslexia—problems with reading—is one of the best known, but there are LDs that affect speech, hearing, handwriting, math, and physical coordination, too. And because so many of these language processing skills are important in different areas of learning, a single LD can cause problems in multiple areas, though it might look different in each area. Once testing and careful observation identify the underlying problem, those differences usually start to make sense.

LDs are incredibly common in kids who have ADHD—in fact, many older lists of LD symptoms included inattentiveness, impulsivity, and hyperactivity, the hallmarks of ADHD. It's true that kids with untreated ADHD struggle with learning, but if ADHD is the only problem, learning gets easier when the ADHD is treated. It's also true that kids with LDs may become anxious or behave inappropriately when faced with yet another school task they know they'll fail. If the only time your son can't sit still is when he's supposed to be doing a writing assignment, he might be struggling with dysgraphia—a learning disability in the physical act of writing—not ADHD.

LDs are also common in children and teens who have bipolar. Formal research studies are under way to measure how prevalent LDs are in these kids, and if certain types are more prevalent than others. Early results suggest that children and teens with bipolar also have problems with attention, working memory, and processing speed, and that these problems are not the result of ADHD being part of the mix.

Many of the children we see have a learning disability of some sort, some mild, some severe. This could be in part because we see many children whose symptoms are extremely complex and severe, but considering how often ADHD occurs with bipolar and how common LDs are with ADHD, we suspect that many kids with bipolar also have an LD or two in the mix.

This is especially important to consider when looking at educational options for your child or teen. Schools do not always recognize that different supports and accommodations are needed for LD and bipolar. (See Chapter 9 for more on educational accommodations.)

Treating LDs is often a combination of tutoring using an individually tailored program and accommodations, such as classroom adjustments, special equipment, and in-class aides.

### Carl: Auditory Processing Disorder

Carl is a tall, skinny seventh-grader who has auditory processing disorder, a learning disability that affects his ability to make sense of what he hears. His hearing acuity is fine—he can hear the sounds—but he has trouble processing those sounds. His teachers have been pretty good about making sure he has written versions of everything, and they know that Carl has a better chance of understanding what they say when there isn't a lot of background noise. He does better when he's calm and knows the routines, too. But sometimes, it's easy to forget that just because Carl can *hear* doesn't mean he can *understand*.

Case in point: A month into seventh grade, Carl's third-period teacher kicked him out of class for misbehaving. She said he refused to sit down where he was supposed to, even though she "told him and told him" why the desks were rearranged and where to sit. Without realizing it, the teacher had automatically given Carl verbal instructions—in a noisy setting, where things were not the same as they had been every day for a month, and where there were no other clues that would let Carl know what he was supposed to do. He was embarrassed as well as confused, and furious that he'd been sent to the principal's office "for no reason at all."

### Samantha: Multiple LDs
Samantha attended a top university on a full academic scholarship and graduated with high honors. She majored in Asian history and minored in theoretical mathematics—even though she has difficulties with writing and has never been able to do basic arithmetic. She almost flunked third grade because she couldn't memorize her times tables, and she was denied entry to a gifted math program because her scores on the written placement exam were very low—despite the fact that she could talk about the same problems and explain them easily and clearly. She uses speech recognition software (and landed her first campus job helping other students use it) and a calculator to work around her learning disabilities.

Chapter 3

## SPINNING STAR

### WHAT BIPOLAR DISORDER
### LOOKS LIKE IN KIDS

*Having bipolar is very very hard, that's for sure. One thing hard to deal with: It makes you feel all the emotions at once, somewhere between meltdown and frozen. Meds help a lot; I don't know what would happen without them. Side effects are annoying but I'm not noticing many. The hardest thing about having bipolar is school. I have a friend with bipolar; we understand what each other is going through. I lose my temper a lot, I have a fast trigger.*

*My advice to other kids is to not completely lose it. Don't obsess or upset yourself about it. Try to learn to live with it, get used to it. Otherwise, you're going to have a bad time.*

LEONARD, AGE ELEVEN, DIAGNOSED AGE FIVE

Why did doctors once think bipolar disorder was so rare in children? Why do experts still argue about how common it is?

Mainly because bipolar disorder doesn't look the same in children as it does in adults.

In adults with Type I bipolar—the classic manic-depression most of us think about when we hear "bipolar"—the person swings from mania to depression and back again. When

Carrie Fisher (Princess Leia of *Star Wars* fame) said that she has two moods, "Roy the manic extrovert and Pam the quiet introvert... Roy decorated my house and Pam has to live in it," and that she's only able to work when she's in between these two extremes, she's describing a classic form of Type I bipolar disorder.

Type II bipolar is similar, but the person doesn't bounce all the way up to full-blown mania. Their "highs" are called *hypomania,* which means "under mania"—higher than an average person's moods, but not as manic as someone with Type I.

In many adults with either Type I or Type II bipolar, the cycles are clear and distinct. One state can last for weeks or months before cycling into the other, and there can be stretches of normal mood states, called *euthymia,* between up and down cycles.

Kids with bipolar may grow up to be adults with one of these two types, but we think they continue to experience what's known in adult psychiatry as *atypical bipolar disorder.* People with atypical bipolar are much more likely to have *mixed states* or *rapid cycling.* A mixed state means experiencing symptoms of mania and depression at the same time. Rapid cycling means switching back and forth between mania and depression very fast. Adults can have mixed states and rapid cycling, too, but mixed states are less common and rapid cycling in an adult means cycling four times or more in a year. To parents, rapid cycling means their child goes through many mood changes in a single day—or hour. Although a sizable number of adults have atypical bipolar, most have Type I or II, but in children and teens, the mixed and complex cycling form is the most common type of bipolar disorder.

Making the picture even more complex is the fact that kids don't behave the same way adults do. (Of course, that's also true of kids and adults who don't have bipolar.) For example, what looks like extreme irritability and stubborn defiance in a six-year-old may in fact be symptoms of mania. In addition, the mood shifts of children with bipolar are often unpredictable and can come out of nowhere; there's no trigger, or there's an extreme reaction to a trigger.

One father described his daughter as a "spinning star." Each point on the star is a different mood or emotional state: explosive rage, extreme irritability, giddiness, depression, and "regular kid." The star spins around, sometimes faster, sometimes slower. It might pause briefly or change direction but there's no way to tell when it will, and there's no way to tell which point of the star you'll see at any given instant. As another parent put it, "I never know who's getting off the school bus."

The good news is that even when the star spins so fast it's a blur, you can identify specific symptoms in your child and, with the help of your child's clinician, determine whether your child's difficulties come from bipolar disorder.

There are two parts to a formal diagnosis of bipolar disorder. The first is simply this: Is your child moody? If so, is the moodiness enough to be a problem?

Kids go through ups and downs all the time. The night before Christmas, the last week of school, a fight with a friend, a really bad day—all kinds of things can affect your child's mood.

So how do we know if "moody" is "mood disorder"?

We look at three things:

*1. Severity (sometimes called intensity).* Moping around the house after school is a pretty ordinary response if your best friend was mean to you at recess today. A four-hour temper tantrum complete with hitting, biting, kicking holes in the walls, and breaking toys is not. It's a big reaction to a small trigger.

Severity includes both how long a symptom lasts (duration) and the level of behavior (its intensity). Generally, a symptom that causes a severe disturbance in one area of life or one that causes a mild or moderate disturbance in several areas is severe enough to contribute to a diagnosis.

2. *Frequency.* Being grouchy because you didn't get a hoped-for toy for your birthday or sad because your favorite teacher is moving are understandable and normal reactions to life's events. Being grouchy or sad many times every day or every week for no reason at all or in response to insignificant events is not. Frequency asks, How often does that symptom or behavior happen? Every day? Many times a day? Is it rare to go more than a day or two without that symptom?

3. *Age-appropriateness.* Toddlers are renowned for the "terrible twos": lots of tantrums and defiance. Short outbursts of anger or frustration and stubbornness are developmentally normal for two- and three-year-olds. In older children, such behavior is cause for concern; the behavior is not developmentally appropriate for a ten-year-old or teenager. And toddler outbursts that are so frequent and severe that they prevent normal toddler activities such as preschool classes and birthday parties aren't developmentally appropriate, either.

Traditionally, the moods of bipolar are divided into two types, depression and mania. You may be used to thinking of these moods as opposites—depression is sad, mania is happy—but there's more to it than that, especially in children and teens.

Kids who are depressed may be lethargic, mopey, or weepy. They may be self-deprecating or suicidal. These are behaviors you expect when someone's depressed. But there's another side to depression: Instead of sad or blue, depressed children and teens may be irritable: whiny, cranky, complaining. With either form of depression, they can also be restless and have trouble concentrating, which is sometimes mistaken for ADHD. They may or may not be able to tell you that they feel sad, blue, or hopeless but may say things like, "I wish I'd never been born," or "I wish I were dead."

In kids, there are two sides to mania, too. One side is the euphoric, elated, high-energy state most people think of when they hear the word "manic." Kids (and adults) in this state can be over-the-top funny—and depending on the kid, the behavior, and the situation, wildly entertaining or thoroughly annoying.

The other side of mania in kids is extreme irritability, which can show up as nastiness, blaming, demanding, whining, or viciousness, punctuated by explosive rages that can be physically abusive, destructive, and dangerous.

Irritability is as important as—and may be more important than—euphoria and sadness in diagnosing bipolar in children and teens. Most families come to us not because they think their child has bipolar but because their child's irritability and explosiveness are so severe that they interfere with the child's ability to function and make life miserable for everyone.

The discovery that extreme irritability is a symptom of mania in children is one of the most important recent breakthroughs in the diagnosis and treatment of bipolar disorder. In the group that Janet Wozniak studied, over half of the kids had irritability and no euphoria, just under half had both, and only 6% had euphoria without significant irritability. Parents whose kids did have euphoria usually brought their child to the clinician because of the irritability, not the euphoria. This shouldn't be a surprise because, generally speaking, irritability is a much more disruptive symptom in a child's life.

Three other important discoveries are also changing our understanding of bipolar. The first is that the severity and type of the bipolar symptoms are the same whether the child has the classic cycling pattern or the more chronic, spinning star course. The second discovery is that the same plus disorders occur with the same frequency regardless of the cycle pattern. And the third is that plus disorders—one, two, or more—are almost always part of the picture. Bipolar rarely appears alone.

These discoveries combined with the realization that bipolar moods in kids don't change in nice neat cycles the way they do in classic adult-onset bipolar has put a whole new spin on how we think of mood disorders. We still look for the telltale signs of depression and mania, but we don't assume they'll show up as single, clearly visible symptoms following a recognizable pattern. We don't assume that one diagnosis will tell the whole story.

No child, bipolar or not, has a week-long stretch of any one mood state, and since most kids with bipolar shift rapidly from one mood state to another and may have several moods happening at once, the traditional diagnostic question of "Did you have a long spell [at least a week] of *this* mood followed by a long spell of *that* mood" doesn't help identify bipolar. So the questions we ask are:

- Is your child in an abnormal mood state most of the time, most days?

- Do you watch her spin through that five-pointed star of rage, irritability, giddiness, depression, and regular kid?

- Does he remind you of Dr. Jekyll and Mr. Hyde?

- Do you feel like you're walking on eggshells all the time to avoid major blowups and meltdowns?

If the answers are no, your child probably doesn't have bipolar disorder—remember, the first part of the formal diagnosis is moodiness frequent and severe enough to cause problems for your child.

If the answers are yes, there may be a mood disorder at work. It might be bipolar—so next, we consider the second part of the formal diagnosis, which looks specifically at mania.

Mania has seven additional symptoms. We remember them as *DIGFAST.*

**D**istractibility
**I**ncreased activity or agitation (high energy)
**G**randiosity
**F**light of ideas or racing thoughts
**A**ctivities with bad outcomes
**S**leep (don't need as much)
**T**alkativeness

Your child might have one or two of these, a mixture of several, or all of them. One might be prominent today, another might be obvious tomorrow. Some might show up when she's irritable but not when she's euphoric. The symptoms you see every day at home might be (and will probably be) entirely different from the ones that surface at school, scout camp, or the shopping mall.

Let's explore these one at a time and see what they look like in real life.

---

Symptoms do NOT have to appear in different settings to count toward a diagnosis!

Many children successfully control their symptoms while at school or in other public places to avoid embarrassment or other social consequences. Some can hold their symptoms in for a long time and only release them once they're in the safer environment of home.

---

## DISTRACTIBILITY

*Peggy is trying hard to pay attention to her teacher, but too many things get in the way. She hears some of what her teacher says, but she also notices the buzz of the fluorescent lights, the stripes of sunlight coming through the window, her teacher's earrings which glinted in the sun as she walked between her desk and the window, other students rustling their papers, and the bright pink ribbon in her left pigtail, which reminds her of the pink dots on her new lunchbox. When the teacher calls on her, Peggy has no idea what the topic is, let alone the question she's supposed to answer. After school, Peggy tries to tell her mom about the cool experiment they did in science class, but her conversation wanders everywhere. When she finally winds down, her mom isn't entirely clear what the experiment was about, though she thinks it had something to do with being outside and the new lunchbox.*

Distraction means difficulty screening out the background clutter of the world while we focus our attention where we want it to be. Kids who are distractible have a hard time staying on task, finishing anything, and attending to detail. They may have trouble telling a story or explaining things because it's difficult for them to tell the difference between what's important and relevant and what's off topic (or way, *way* off topic). Their brain is either zipping off into the next shiny thing (zing-zing-zing, never able to stop long enough to do anything) or is inundated with the awareness of everything all at once, regardless of how relevant any of it is.

If you're thinking this sounds a lot like ADHD, you're right; even the formal descriptions of distractibility in mania and ADHD in the DSM-IV are the same. So how do we know which we're dealing with?

First, distractibility alone, no matter how severe, is not enough to diagnose either mania or ADHD. For mania, we need an abnormal mood state plus at least three of the seven major symptoms. For ADHD, we need six of its nine diagnostic criteria, impulsivity, for example.

Second, even then, we may not know whether mania or ADHD—or both—is causing the distractibility. It isn't unusual to identify all the symptoms of ADHD first, and then ask: Is there a mood disorder, too? Or looking at it another way, if you have a moody ADHD child, is that really mania? Or is the moodiness caused by something else—perhaps the low frustration tolerance common in ADHD or a bad reaction to medication?

Remember that mood disorder is the first part of identifying bipolar. If your child is distractible but there's no sign of fluctuating moods causing problems in her life, then it probably isn't bipolar. If there are signs of fluctuating moods and she's distractible, her distractibility might be a symptom of mania—but considering how common bipolar plus ADHD is, the distractibility could easily be from both.

By the way, common clinical lore says that distractibility from ADHD is constant and distractibility from mania changes or cycles like moods do. Whether or not this is true, in real life, it's not useful for diagnosing. A child with ADHD can have a great attention span when engaged in something he loves (video games, for example) and a child with mania may be distractible most of the time because he has the spinning star pattern.

## INCREASED ACTIVITY, AGITATION, OR ENERGY

*Melissa sits cross-legged on her bedroom floor, intently folding colorful squares of paper into precise origami figures. She has decided to make three origamis for everyone in her class, including the teacher. It is two o'clock in the morning; her parents have given up trying to get her to quit for the night. She absolutely will not be deterred. Despite being exhausted, she carefully folds each sheet, discarding any that do not meet her exacting standards.*

*Ten-year-old Isaiah decided to start a business. Soon, everything in his world revolved around the business idea. He wrote and rewrote elaborate plans. He pestered nonstop for materials to make the products he wanted to sell in the front yard. He had no interest in doing anything unless it somehow connected to this project.*

*Kenny's latest project is an enormous mural that's supposed to be done in time for the high school homecoming game. He's also working on a stone sculpture for extra credit in art; has convinced the dance committee to redo all the decorations (and promised to help); and has persuaded the drama club to let him direct a play he's writing. He practically crackles with energy, pacing, gesturing, holding three conversations at once.*

Melissa, Isaiah, and Kenny are all showing increased goal-directed activity, the "I" of DIGFAST.

Some parents describe this symptom as "manic mission mode." Their son or daughter gets an idea about doing something and then focuses on that to the exclusion of all else. Sometimes, it's a great idea and the result is amazingly productive. Sometimes, it's silly, strange, or useless; they're spinning their wheels and can't get out of this fixated state to function at school or go to sleep.

In casual conversation, Melissa's mom might say her daughter's obsessed with origami, and Isaiah's dad might talk about his son's obsession with business—but are their children's intense interests really obsessive-compulsive disorder? A symptom of mania? Or something else?

Here's another place where identifying bipolar and bipolar plus can be tricky.

There are least four types of fixated behavior:

*Obsessive-compulsive disorder* (OCD)—true obsessions;
*Manic mission mode*—increased goal-directed activity;
*Asperger's syndrome*—restricted number of interests, difficulty shifting attention smoothly and making transitions from one activity to another;
*Hyperfocus associated with ADHD*—ability to sustain intense concentration on a high-interest activity for an extended stretch of time.

These behaviors can mimic each other, making it hard to sort out why a child is fixated on a particular thing.

So, parents and clinicians look at what else is going on. What else does Melissa do? If she has other symptoms of OCD, for example, counting things and anxiety about germs, then her three-origami-per-classmate project may have its roots in OCD. If folding paper is enjoyable and comforting, she knows more than anyone cares to know about origami, and she has difficulty in social interactions, Melissa's fixation on origami might be part of Asperger's syndrome. Depending on whether there are other symptoms of a mood disorder, the fixation might be a symptom of mania. And of course, Melissa's origami might be a symptom of all three conditions at the same time.

Kenny, our super-active high school artist, is also showing increased goal-directed activity. Instead of being fixated on one specific idea or project, he's overextended in lots of activities and is staying awake through the night to execute his plans. He's on the go continually and looks like a master of multitasking—but he adds new projects without considering whether or not he can finish them. He barges into conversations, calls friends at all hours, and is clueless about why anyone would be upset with him.

Jumping from project to project, interrupting and intruding, and being physically restless: These can be symptoms of mania—and of ADHD. Just like distractibility, "increased activity" can stem from bipolar, ADHD, or both.

## GRANDIOSITY

*Four-year-old Tommy disappeared from his house. The police and neighbors were still searching for him at nightfall—five hours later— when he wandered back. His frantic parents asked him where he'd been. "I'm camping out," Tommy said. "I just came back to get my pillow." His parents and a police officer followed Tommy into the wooded area bordering their subdivision to his "campsite." He did have pretty much everything he needed; he knew what to take thanks to a TV show he'd seen that morning. It didn't occur to him that he needed permission from his parents along with everything else. Is this grandiosity? ADHD impulsivity? Or an adventurous four-year-old?*

*Josh is standing on the top step of the ladder, hammer firmly in hand. He looks across the roof to where two men are pounding nails into new shingles. "Hey," he shouts. "You need to leave now. I am going to do this work, not you." If Josh is three, is this grandiosity? If he's ten? If he's seventeen?*

*Leah is sixteen. She's a good driver; she'd aced driver's ed, gotten her license on her first try, and had never had an accident or ticket. Last week, she took her mother's car in the middle of the night and headed west. When her mother finally got her home again and asked where she thought she was going, Leah told her, "To Hollywood, to start my movie career without you in my way." Is this grandiosity? Ambition? Naiveté?*

Grandiosity is inflated self-esteem, the belief that you are bigger, better, stronger, prettier, smarter than others when in reality, you're not.

It is one of the symptoms of mania—and it's a common trait of children, part of normal development. It isn't easy to distinguish abnormal grandiosity. As with other symptoms, we look for patterns: severity, frequency, and age-appropriateness, plus the company it keeps—what other symptoms does your child have?

The occasional playground scuffle is probably not the result of grandiosity, nor is the every now and again declaration of being smarter than the teacher. But when a child is so thoroughly convinced that he's tougher than everybody that he picks fights with the big kids and gets beat up every day, grandiosity is likely part of the problem. The teen who thinks he's smarter than everyone at school, continually argues with and insults the teacher, and refuses to do his schoolwork because "the teacher's an idiot" has stepped beyond ordinary adolescent arrogance.

Grandiose behaviors can be charming or cute—when your

nine-year-old sends her movie ideas to Spielberg, for example, or your toddler stomps his foot and refuses to do as he's told. It's not so cute when your seventeen-year-old drives to Washington, DC, on a moment's notice because he thinks he can change the vote in Congress. Grandiosity's even worse when it slides into oppositional defiant disorder (ODD).

Almost all kids with bipolar have some level of ODD. Ongoing research with the bipolar plus ODD combination is confirming that there are different types of ODD, one of which has the distinct grandiose flavor seen in mania.

Kids with grandiosity and ODD show flagrant or outrageous disregard for authority. At home, they rule the roost—not because their parents are pushovers, but because there is no reasoning with them. They belittle their parents, feel put-upon whenever they're challenged, and defy authority at every turn.

## FLIGHT OF IDEAS AND RACING THOUGHTS

*Jessica has been talking nonstop for hours. She bounces from topic to topic, sometimes switching in midsentence, and despite her dad's prompting to "slow down, back up, now tell me the point," even she loses track of what she's trying to say. She quiets down at bedtime but complains that she can't get to sleep because her brain won't turn off.*

Excessive talkativeness (the "T" of DIGFAST, see below) is often the only external clue that your son or daughter is experiencing flight of ideas (FOI). In FOI, the brain bounces from topic to topic, never staying on anything very long. The bouncing around can be so fast that speech becomes garbled—disorganized, incoherent, and unintelligible.

Racing thoughts are similar to FOI and sometimes more difficult to recognize, because your child might be feeling this phenomenon but not talking about it. Racing thoughts are thoughts that flood in so fast that your child might not be able to talk about them because there's no way to keep up. Some kids say they wish they could "turn their brains down." They might blurt things out so they don't lose a particular thought.

Racing thoughts can overlap and are sometimes difficult to distinguish from anxiety. They can magnify the anxiety, too, when anxious thoughts become racing thoughts and flood the child with anxiety.

## ACTIVITIES WITH BAD OUTCOMES

*Jesse has a bad case of the giggles. "Poopyhead," he says, giggling. "Poopy poopy poopyhead." His mother scowls at him; he grins and settles down for a minute—but only a minute—while she continues her conversation. Then he launches enthusiastically into a story he's told dozens of times, one of his favorites. His mom tries to redirect him but he rattles on until he gleefully reaches the punch line of the story about his best friend—"And he pooped on the floor." Jesse's mom sighs; she knows at thirteen, he's way too old for potty humor, and this is definitely over the top.*

*Sean's first-grade teacher notices he's wriggling in his chair again. It isn't general fidgeting or ADHD. He's masturbating, which a lot of kids do, especially when they're young and still learning appropriate social behavior, but Sean does this a lot. Yesterday, she caught him exposing himself on the playground again. He's always trying to touch the private parts of other kids or look under their clothes, and she's never seen a kid so intent on "playing doctor." To Sean's teacher, these behaviors can mean only one thing. She's put in a call to social services about suspected sexual abuse.*

*Cory began surfing porn sites on the Internet when he was thirteen. He spends hours online every night, most of it after his parents have gone to bed. Much to his parents' surprise and dismay, he has a whole network of "friends" online, and he's convinced several kids from school to check out his favorite sites.*

*Kirsten is a tall, slender fifteen-year-old. She dresses in the latest styles and expertly applies her makeup every morning before school. Today, she's wearing a low-cut midriff-baring knit top that shows off the cleavage from her new lace push-up bra. Her skirt is short, low-slung, bright red, and tight. Her shoes are new; strappy black sandals with three-inch heels that she's been bugging her mom to buy for weeks. Her parents call her a shopaholic and are on her case about her risqué outfits. They argue all the time about how much money she spends. Kirsten doesn't care; she's convinced she looks good. She tells others that she's sure it's worth it, because she's leaving any day now for California to be a movie star. She met a guy when she was partying who claims that he can make it happen.*

Everybody makes mistakes; it's part of being human. For most of us, learning that some activities (drinking too much or blowing an entire paycheck on clothes, for example) result in unpleasant consequences leads to better judgment the next time around. For kids with mania, that isn't necessarily true. Even a child who understands the consequences and has shown good judgment in the past may lose those abilities during a manic episode.

And, as with many other symptoms we've talked about, it may be challenging to tease out psychiatric symptoms from intense-but-still-normal behavior. Are your teen's ambitions for fame and glory grounded in youthful optimism and inexperience? Or the grandiosity and mission mode of mania? Some kids experiment with drugs and alcohol, which impacts their judgment even more; is the drug abuse its own problem or is it part of mania—or both?

If your child is pursuing activities that are inappropriate and potentially harmful despite the risks and negative consequences, you've got a kid exhibiting the "A" of DIGFAST: activities with bad outcomes.

At their worst, these actions can lead to jail and substance abuse, two of the three scariest risks for kids with bipolar (the third is suicide).

Often, you'll see other elements of mania in this symptom, especially grandiosity (I'll never get caught, I'm better than everybody, the cops are fools, the law doesn't apply to me) and increased activity or mission mode (unrelenting requests for a new toy, for example), as well as the lack of insight common in all phases of bipolar (It's all your fault, the problem is you, there's nothing wrong with me, you never let me do what I want).

Of the wide range of behaviors that might show up as activities with bad outcomes, two—hypersexuality and spending— are especially important, both because they're common and because they're often misinterpreted or misunderstood.

## HYPERSEXUALITY

Is your child hypersexual?

If you're like many of the parents we see, your automatic response is, "No, of course not!"

*Hypersexuality* does *not* mean "having sex." A better question to ask is, "Does your child do things, say things, or have an interest in sexual matters that are inappropriate for your child's age?"

Hypersexual behaviors range from potty humor, running around naked, and inappropriate touching to porn addictions, promiscuity, and prostitution.

Not all "sexual" behaviors are "hypersexual." Preschoolers are fascinated with bodies; that's part of normal development. A toddler who pulls off all her clothes in the middle of the park may be too hot, hate the scratchy tag in her T-shirt, or be asserting her independence. Little girls try out Mom's makeup; middle school boys discover dirty jokes.

Confusing the issue even more is that we live in a sexually saturated society. Ads glorify sexy fashions for younger and younger buyers, TV shows are more explicit, pornography is easily available. Comments, clothes, and behaviors that would have been shocking in young people fifty years ago are practically mainstream in much of today's American society.

That said, most kids are easily redirected when it comes to what's appropriate and private. Once beyond toddlerhood, most kids don't touch other people's private parts. Potty humor and dirty jokes are relegated to sanctioned places (locker rooms, late-night comedy shows), not shared at the dinner table.

So when we're trying to identify hypersexual behavior, we're looking at the same three clues we use for other behaviors: severity, frequency, and age-appropriateness. Which brings us back to our earlier question: Does your child do or say things or have an interest in sexual matters inappropriate for his or her age? If the answer is yes, you may be observing hypersexual behavior.

By itself, hypersexuality does not equal bipolar disorder—your child must have the severe moodiness that is the first part of any bipolar diagnosis as well as other symptoms of mania.

### Hypersexuality or Sexual Abuse?

It's the phone call—or accusation—every parent dreads: The school is convinced your child is the victim of sexual abuse. The Department of Social Services has been notified and your family is about to be put under the microscope.

The effects of sexual trauma have been studied for a long time. High-profile cases, the efforts of parents, advocates, and victims' rights groups, and mainstream media reports have done a great job of raising public awareness of this very real problem. On the whole, that's good; children who are sexually traumatized need to be recognized and helped, and their perpetrators need to be found and dealt with.

Mania in children, including hypersexuality, is a much newer concept. Even when other symptoms of mania or bipolar disorder are present, most clinicians, counselors, and teachers assume that all sexual acting out is the result of abuse. Hypersexuality, a symptom of mania, is almost always overlooked as a potential cause of sexually inappropriate behavior.

*Hypersexuality is not equivalent to evidence of abuse.* It can and does happen as a direct result of mania.

If you—or the doctor, school, or other authority—don't consider mania as a possible cause for a child's sexually inappropriate behavior, you're not just in danger of barking up the wrong tree, you may be looking in the wrong forest.

Kids who are hypersexual are at higher risk of sexual abuse because the nature of their illness can put them in harm's way. For example, if a hypersexual young boy is trying to engage other children his age in sexual activities, he is more likely to be noticed by an adult pedophile. It is entirely possible that both problems—mania and sexual trauma—are driving the hypersexual behavior.

So how do we tell if the behavior is from hypersexuality, trauma, or both?

Kids who have been sexually traumatized may act out sexually, but their behavior tends to be more specific and reflects the abuse they've experienced. For example, a young child playing with dolls might show the dolls having sex, with a running commentary that includes specific language and physical details.

Kids who are hypersexual and sexually inexperienced won't know that level of detail, and their hypersexuality will occur across a broader spectrum of behaviors.

Another clue to the "is it abuse or is it mania" question is found in examining the other symptoms the child has.

Some sexually traumatized children have flashbacks and intrusive thoughts related to sex in general or to the specific abuse they experienced. These thoughts, which are part of the anxiety disorder post-traumatic stress disorder (PTSD), can overwhelm the child in much the same way that the flight of ideas (FOI) and racing thoughts of mania can. In mania's FOI, the ideas crowd and bounce around from topic to topic and don't repeat. This frantic jumble might make your child frustrated because he can't latch onto an idea long enough to communicate or make it difficult to fall asleep because his brain is "busy," but it usually won't make him anxious or afraid. Racing thoughts might aggravate anxiety, if your child also has an anxiety disorder—and if the anxiety is PTSD, your child may be experiencing both intrusive thoughts and mania's racing thoughts.

Some victims of sexual abuse erupt in rages that look a lot like the rages and extreme irritability we see in mania—so much so that if you're looking only at the rage storms and acting out, you might not be able to tell the difference. It's important to remember that one symptom by itself isn't enough to make a diagnosis. We must look at all the criteria for bipolar, from "Part A: Is your child moody?" through every point of the spinning star. If your child's symptoms meet the criteria for bipolar, that's the diagnosis, whether or not there has been sexual trauma.

We also hunt for other clues—family history, patterns, and things that trigger behaviors— to help identify what is driving the behavior. Behaviors driven by sexual abuse, other trauma, or other plus disorders tend to have a more consistent pattern; a particular behavior, nasty temper tantrums, for example, is consistently triggered by the same or similar things. Behaviors driven by mania are more "all over"; you see the behavior in different settings and different situations, initiated by different triggers or arising out of the blue, for no apparent reason.

While mania can lead in some cases to trauma, trauma may trigger or set the stage for mania or depression. It's important to recognize whether a child's inappropriate behavior is hypersexuality driven by mania, sexual acting out stemming from sexual trauma, or both because treatment plans differ. Treatment for one won't work for the other and might worsen it. In addition to therapy and protection from the perpetrator, treatment for kids with PTSD often includes a class of medications known as SSRIs *(selective serotonin reuptake inhibitors)*, which can make mania worse. (For more on treatment, see Chapter 7.)

## SPENDING

Adults with this symptom of mania overspend, go into debt, get involved in crazy business schemes, and buy loads of stuff they don't need. Fortunes have been won—and lost—during manic episodes.

Most kids don't have access to that kind of capital, but it doesn't make the problem any easier.

They're shopaholics, continually nagging their parents for something new. When they finally wear down Mom or Dad and get the new toy or sweater or gadget, it doesn't bring them joy or delight; immediately and continually, they're pestering for something new. Often, no matter what you try, you won't be able to sidetrack these kids from their desire to buy whatever new thing they've focused on. This intense focus can overlap with manic mission mode ("I"), grandiosity ("G"), and illegal behaviors like shoplifting or other types of stealing.

For example, Amanda, a petite seven-year-old, was adamant about getting a Louis Vuitton pocketbook. We asked her how she even knew what a Louis Vuitton pocketbook was and she said, "Everybody knows! I have to have it." She was extremely demanding; as far as she was concerned, she needed the designer purse. She didn't—and couldn't, in her mania—see it as a luxury.

Other kids aren't focused on spending but are foolish with their money. They give all their money (or toys) away, or buy candy and ice cream for everybody. The hole their money burns in their pockets is so big that it becomes a family problem.

## SLEEP (DECREASED NEED FOR)

*Danica starts getting silly every evening after supper. As the rest of her family is winding down from the day, Danica is winding up. Her goofy, giddy behavior ranges from funny and entertaining to annoying. She pours her restlessness into dance and gymnastics. She's literally cartwheeled across her room for hours every night this week.*

*In the mornings, she's almost impossible to awaken. She's groggy and grouchy and refuses to get out of bed. It's not quite as bad on mornings when she doesn't have to go to school, but it still takes her a long time to wake up.*

About one-third of the kids with bipolar have a decreased need for sleep. "Decreased need for sleep" does *not* mean:

- A night owl whose internal clock is set for a later bedtime and later start in the morning

- Staying up until three a.m., getting up on time for breakfast, and being tired all day

- Staying up until three a.m. and sleeping until noon every weekend

"Decreased need for sleep" *does* mean that they function with high energy on less, little, or no sleep.

Kids with bipolar often have other problems related to sleep or sleep cycles in addition to this decreased need for sleep.

Our internal sense of when to wake up and when to fall asleep is governed by our circadian rhythm. The circadian rhythm is our internal clock, and its natural rhythm—the time it takes to go through one full cycle—is about twenty-five hours. The clock is reset every day by external cues such as sunrise.

There are individual variations in circadian rhythms. Whether you're a lark (early riser) or an owl (slower to get going in the morning) depends on your particular circadian rhythm. Most people are diurnal—their circadian rhythm is set for them to wake up in the morning, stay awake during the day, and sleep at night.

Adolescence shifts the circadian rhythm so that it's more nocturnal. The "time for sleep" signal happens later at night, and you don't feel like going to sleep until much later than you normally would. Teens want to be up later because of this shift and if they have bipolar disorder, they may need less sleep overall, which throws their sleep cycle off even more.

On the morning side of the sleep equation, teens have an incredibly difficult time waking up, even when they do get to sleep early enough, and this may be worse with bipolar disorder. Lots of teens have an exaggerated version of the "up-late-sleep-in" pattern of typical teenagers. Add bipolar to the mix and the result is a huge problem with the necessary daily activity of waking up in time for school.

Medications used to treat bipolar disorder also affect sleep cycles, though the specific impact a medication has varies from child to child. Most of the time, meds help the child sleep better, but they don't solve the "hard to wake up" problem and may make it worse.

School can also aggravate the morning wake-up challenge. A lot of kids cope at school, keeping the symptoms under control once they're there. This takes a tremendous amount of energy and effort on their part, and there's continual worry that they'll "lose it" in front of everybody. Little wonder that waking up on school days is a harder battle than waking up on weekends.

Other symptoms of bipolar can interfere with sleep, too. For example, kids with racing thoughts might complain that they can't sleep because their brain won't "turn off" or "quiet down." Kids in mission mode (increased activity/agitation) won't sleep because they're consumed by their activity.

Plus disorders cause problems, too. Kids with ADHD may have a tough time settling down. Kids with anxiety disorders may refuse to sleep unless Mom or Dad stays in the room. Those who have had traumatic experiences may have bad dreams.

There has been some speculation that children with bipolar have problems both getting to sleep and resting well during sleep because they have night terrors and gruesome dreams, but there is no research that supports this. Some kids, possibly more boys than girls, imagine gruesome and gory stuff when they're awake, and some have nightmares and night terrors, but neither of these is a primary symptom of bipolar. The problems with sleep, from decreased need to disrupted circadian rhythms, are much more complex than the aftereffects of vivid nightmares.

Aggravating the situation is that not only can mania bring a decreased need for sleep, sleep deprivation regardless of the cause can make the mood symptoms of bipolar worse. Not enough sleep can be both a symptom and a cause.

## TALKATIVENESS

*Nicky is a nonstop talker. He talks when he's happy and excited; he talks when he's crabby and irritable. He talks whether it's his turn or not, and he keeps talking long after anyone trying to listen is lost or overwhelmed. Sometimes, the things he says don't make sense; the words and ideas are jumbled, or he leapfrogs from one story to another with no warning. His speech is rapid-fire, his words tumbling out like floodwaters rushing over a dam.*

The talkativeness of mania is similar to flight of ideas (FOI) and racing thoughts. FOI and racing thoughts may be entirely internal—your child's thoughts are bouncing all over the map or they're flooding in too fast to track, but you don't know that's what's going on because you're not a mind reader. Talkativeness is the external evidence—your little chatterbox's language reflects what's going on with her thoughts.

This rapid-fire, excessive talking is called *pressured speech.* There's a sense of urgency, of needing to get the words out *now.* It's hard to interrupt, and the child can't sense the social cues that would tell her she's overstepped boundaries or lost her audience.

You've probably heard pressured speech even if you've never been near anyone with bipolar disorder. It's the normal speaking style of many speakers and others who are enthusiastic or just trying to get through a lot of material in a short time. In fact, it's the speaking style of one of this book's authors (we'll let you guess who), which is why we like to use this symptom as a reminder that one symptom does not equal a diagnosis.

There are two plus disorders that may include excessive talkativeness. The one that's most similar to pressured speech is the impulsive, distractible ADHD chatterbox. In fact, there may not be *any* difference between the pressured speech of mania and the talkativeness of ADHD. We have to rely on other symptoms to help us identify if it's bipolar, ADHD, both, or neither.

The talkativeness of kids with Asperger's syndrome is usually quite different from the talkativeness of mania or ADHD. The speaking style of a child with Asperger's isn't pressured or rapid-fire, though it may be unusual in tone or inflection. A child with Asperger's won't jump from topic to topic, either; he'll stay on track (typically a very narrow track), talking about his particular passionate interest.

The stories we've shared in this chapter each emphasize a particular symptom so it's easier to understand and recognize the symptom, but remember, one symptom alone is not enough to diagnose bipolar disorder or any of the plus disorders. This doesn't mean the symptom isn't a problem for your child, only that by itself, the symptom won't meet the requirements for diagnosis.

Although one symptom isn't enough for a diagnosis, your child doesn't have to have all of the symptoms, either. The symptoms she does have can be at different levels of severity and frequency. Some might wax and wane. Some might be a problem only at home or only during a certain time of day. Others might be completely unpredictable.

The severity of bipolar disorder, like any illness, varies from person to person. We often describe this variation as the bipolar spectrum. At one end of the spectrum are children who are extremely ill, with many severe and frequent symptoms. At the other end of the spectrum are children with fewer and milder, occasionally problematic, symptoms. Their symptoms aren't severe enough to justify a diagnosis of bipolar, but they're "on the bipolar spectrum."

*Chapter 4*

# THE WHOSE-FAULT PITFALL

## WHAT CAUSES BIPOLAR DISORDER?

Like many of the parents who come to us for help, you may feel a deep sense of shame. You may think you've failed your child, because nothing you do works. Chances are, you've gotten plenty of "advice" that says your child's problems are your fault.

By now, you've been accused of being too lenient, too strict, too inconsistent. You've been told that your child has problems because Mom is mentally ill or at least serving the wrong food, or because Dad is absent, abusive, or indulgent. You've probably been blamed by friends and relatives and by professionals—teachers, psychotherapists, physicians—both directly and indirectly. You and your spouse may be blaming each other, too.

It's easy to fall into the "whose-fault" pitfall. If you were a good parent, so the thinking goes, you'd have a good child.

But the truth is that bad parenting has nothing to do with bipolar disorder. It doesn't cause it, and being a better parent won't cure it.

If bad parenting doesn't cause bipolar disorder, what does?

The very short answer: We don't know yet.

The slightly longer answer: A physically based brain malfunction short-circuits some thoughts and feelings. It is an *illness* caused by a *physical organ* (the brain). It is not a character fault or the result of faulty parenting.

If your heart isn't working right, your lips might turn blue or you might get out of breath or have horrible pain. The same relationship exists between the brain and behavior or mood problems. All thinking and feeling come from the brain. The behavior and moods that we observe (or feel) are the outward signs of those thoughts and feelings. If the brain isn't working right, then the thoughts and feelings that it generates won't be right, either.

Figuring out what causes the brain malfunction that results in bipolar disorder is especially challenging because not everyone has identical symptoms, and even people with the same symptoms could have different underlying "causes" or "illnesses." The same way that three people vomiting might have three different illnesses, say a concussion, food poisoning, and the flu, people with similarly appearing bipolar disorder could have different genetic or brain causes. By the same token, three people may have the very same flu virus, but one has a vicious headache, the other has body aches, and the third a high fever. When the illness begins, how severe the symptoms are, and how symptoms change over time are different, too. Is the bipolar disorder that appears in a very young child caused by the same thing as the bipolar disorder that first appears in adulthood? Do manic irritability and rage storms stem from the same cause as manic euphoria and sleepless nights? Are the causes the same in different children?

We diagnose bipolar disorder by clinical observation: We add our observations of your child's behavior to your (and your child's) observations and, based on published criteria and our clinical experience, we make a diagnosis. The diagnosis is our best attempt at describing a group of symptoms that often show up together. Most likely, what we are really describing is a heterogeneous illness: Bipolar is the big category, but it includes many subtypes. Different subtypes might have different causes or combinations of causes.

In searching for causes, we're also searching for clues that tell us how likely it is that someone might develop bipolar, help us provide faster and more precise diagnosis, and lead to more effective treatment. Although research has not yet revealed all the details of how brains affected by bipolar disorder work (or misfire), we have learned a lot about how to help people while the research into causes continues.

Looking for the causes of bipolar takes us into three areas: genetics, brain cell communication, and the physical structure of the brain.

## GENETICS

Any psychiatric problem is an interplay of biology and environment, what many people call *nature* and *nurture*.

We often think of nature as what we're born with—our inborn strengths and weaknesses. These stem from our genetic makeup, the genes encoded in our DNA that control our physical appearance and whether we're left- or right-handed, for example. Our unique genetic mix is what makes us unique individuals.

Nurture is much more than parenting skills. It includes every environmental factor your child has ever been exposed to from the moment of conception, including blood flow through the placenta, viruses, toxins in food and air, birth trauma, and blind chance.

Looking at family histories—which relatives have (or had) bipolar or other things that might be connected to bipolar (the plus disorders, other mental illnesses, substance abuse, or alcoholism, for example)—clearly shows that genetics plays a role in bipolar disorder. About 40% of the children we see have one or more close relatives with the illness. But for the other 60%, there are no relatives or only distant relatives with bipolar disorder. Most parents of kids with bipolar don't have bipolar themselves, and in most families, their other children don't have the illness. In families where a parent has bipolar, there's about a one in five chance that a child will develop bipolar, but there's a greater chance of developing depression. Identical twins have identical genes, but when one twin has bipolar, the other one develops the illness only 60% of the time, and their symptoms may be quite different. This is true whether the twins grew up together in the same household or if they were raised by different sets of parents worlds apart.

If bipolar is inherited, why doesn't everyone have the same symptoms? the same age of onset and the same severity? the same reaction to medication? These things vary within a group of relatives as well as between unrelated individuals and between kids who are in similar environments and those who are in completely different situations—but there are still enough similarities that we can define bipolar as a reasonably consistent set of symptoms. What's going on?

The variability suggests that bipolar disorder is *polygenetic,* or controlled by different genes.

A gene is a segment of DNA that carries the code for a particular trait. In the simplest genetic case, if you have that gene, you'll have the trait. When a gene is broken, the trait it codes for will be broken, too. "Broken" means the gene might be missing, there might be a problem with its on-off switches, or it might have an error in its code so that the protein it makes is defective, resulting in a particular symptom or behavior.

These changes, or mutations, in the genes might be the ones you inherited from your parents, could be the result of something gone wrong in the womb, or could be pure happenstance, part of the normal variation that occurs when cells divide and grow. Whether these changes lead to behavioral issues or symptoms could also involve environmental influences: something as uncontrollable as exposure to a virus or as pronounced as extended severe trauma.

The genetic impact of bipolar most likely results from several genes, not just one. Symptoms could occur because a gene or set of genes directly responsible for some part of brain structure or brain functioning is damaged, so the structure can't form properly or the brain can't do certain tasks correctly or at all. The number of genes affected determines your vulnerability; the more genes that are affected, the greater your chances of developing bipolar.

Imagine that all the possible variations of the genes involved in bipolar and the plus disorders are a deck of playing cards. Each of us is dealt a hand from that deck. Some people get a great hand—aces and kings; they're so resilient, they'll be fine even if they experience severe trauma. Others aren't so lucky—low, mismatched cards; no matter how ideal their environment is, they'll still develop bipolar. Most of us hold cards that are somewhere in between those two extremes. We have some high cards that protect us, some low cards that make us more vulnerable, and some cards in the middle that might tip the balance one way or the other depending on what life brings.

Polygenetics helps explain why someone may develop bipolar disorder even when there's no family history of the illness. With any well-shuffled deck, there's a lot of random chance that determines what cards are dealt each time around. A low card or two might not have any visible effect. It's only when, by luck of the draw, a hand has the unlucky combination of cards that bipolar surfaces.

When scientists began searching for the genes involved in bipolar, they looked at groups of adults diagnosed as bipolar. Some had childhood onset, some adult onset, and each had a variety of symptoms and plus disorders. These scientists may have inadvertently lumped different but related illnesses together, making it hard to find the particular unlucky cards responsible for any specific illness or subtype.

Over time, research has focused on specific subtypes of bipolar that are easy to identify, track, and measure. Instead of trying to figure out the genetics by looking at a group of many types of bipolar, we examine, for example, only those with early childhood onset or those that occur with ADHD. These specific groups may all be holding similar "unlucky cards" (genes responsible for the disorder). Then we can focus in even more closely, looking at those with bipolar plus family history, or those with bipolar plus certain cognitive features. We can even look for smaller traits that can be measured, such as those with smaller amygdalae (a part of the brain), brain imaging findings, or levels of hormones, enzymes, and chemicals in the brain and bloodstream. Such traits might be present in non-bipolar relatives as well, giving us clues about what makes up a "good hand." When we get down to traits this small, we're studying *endophenotypes*—the physical outcomes our genes produce that are too small to see directly, but are key steps in the development of the illness we call bipolar.

The idea behind this is that while the entire bipolar illness results from many genes, endophenotypes result from just a few of those genes. As we identify genes for a particular endophenotype, we'll begin to understand the genetics for the entire bipolar spectrum, ultimately identifying all the genes that can be involved in bipolar. Identifying endophenotypes may also lead to markers that can tell us who is at risk, what to do to help prevent the onset of bipolar, and what kind of treatment will be most effective for an individual.

Studying endophenotypes will help identify which genes are involved, but that isn't the whole story. We also want to know what is different about those genes. What is the "two of clubs" doing differently than the "king of diamonds"? If we know this, it may also help us predict the development of bipolar and identify better treatment.

For example, one possible difference is that genes involved in bipolar disorder turn on or off at the wrong time. Researchers in *epigenetics* study what activates and deactivates a gene—the gene's on-off switch—and what happens when a particular gene is turned on or off.

When a gene is activated or turned on, it produces the protein encoded in its DNA. When it's deactivated, it stops producing the protein. It's easy to see that turning a gene on or off at the wrong time could cause a problem, but it leads to another question: What flips the gene's switch?

We once assumed that a gene was like a lamp with a light switch. Turn the switch on and the lamp turns on; turn the switch off and the lamp turns off. Ten genes were like ten lamps, each lamp with its own switch, separate from the other lamps. As long as the lamps were hooked up to the electricity, it didn't matter whether they were inside or outside, close together or scattered around different rooms, or whether any of the other lamps were on. If the switch for a particular lamp was "on," the lamp controlled by that switch was on.

As we've started to look carefully at clusters of genes, endophenotypes, and epigenetics, we've discovered that genes are influenced by each other, and they are influenced by their environment.

Using our light switch example, this means that our ability to turn a lamp on or off depends on more than its switch. It might depend on where the lamp is (if it's outside on a sunny day, it won't turn on even if the switch is "on"), whether the other lamps are on (perhaps your lamp won't shine unless some of the others are turned off), and how close it is to other lamps.

If your lightbulb's broken and won't turn on at all, maybe that's not a problem, because nine other lamps are working just fine. Maybe they shine a little brighter to make up for the broken lamp. If your lamp has a loose wire, perhaps it will turn on only after you flip the switch several times, and once on, it interferes with the other lamps; they can't shine as brightly. And if the switch is broken, your lamp will be stuck either on or off.

Here, on the molecular and genetic level (where it ought to be a lot simpler than when we were looking at the whole tangle of bipolar symptoms), we begin to understand how complex the genetics of bipolar disorder can be. Bipolar disorder isn't just the sum of all the genes; it's the sum of the genes directly involved, plus the influence of other genes, plus the influence of the environment from the molecular level on up on both directly involved genes and influencing genes. And it doesn't stop there; the endophenotypes that result from the activated genes become part of the environment and add their influences, so there's continuing feedback to the system.

The number of possible combinations is stunning. With so many potential pitfalls, it's amazing that our brains work as well as they do—and not surprising that there is so much variation.


## GENETICS AND THE PLUS DISORDERS

The plus disorders—ADHD, anxiety, depression, ODD, and CD—have complex genetics, too. Age of onset, type and severity of symptoms, responses to treatment, and family histories all point to polygenetics. The similarity and outright overlap of symptoms among these disorders and with bipolar suggests that some of the same genes and gene combinations are probably involved—hyperactivity in bipolar and ADHD may stem from the same genes, for example, or the ADHD that occurs with bipolar might be different from the ADHD that occurs alone. The severity of symptoms in one disorder may be influenced by the genes that underlie another. And the fact that these disorders occur so often alongside bipolar makes it likely that many of the affected genes are located near each other on a chromosome; they're more likely to be inherited together as a group.

## LOOKING FOR CAUSES, FINDING SOLUTIONS

As recently as 1997, child psychiatry experts were debating whether children who had the symptoms of bipolar really had bipolar, or if they had a severe variant of ADHD. We now know that kids do, in fact, develop bipolar—and they often have ADHD, too.

Research exploring what causes these disorders may eventually help us diagnose them more accurately, which is especially important for treatment. Treating bipolar as if it is ADHD usually makes the bipolar worse. Treating ADHD as if it is bipolar doesn't work well, either.

In 2006, Moore, Biederman, Wozniak, and others used proton magnetic resonance spectroscopy (H-MRS) to measure the relative amounts of several substances in a specific region of the brain in three groups of children and adolescents. One group had ADHD only; one group had bipolar disorder plus ADHD; and one group had no psychiatric illness.

Their results showed significant differences between the three groups. These differences added more evidence supporting current theories about what causes ADHD and might, if confirmed, be used to differentiate between kids who have ADHD with and without bipolar. The results also provided clues to explain why lithium and valproate (both medications used to treat bipolar) don't work as well for kids who have bipolar plus ADHD.

## CELL-TO-CELL COMMUNICATION:
## NEURONS AND NEUROTRANSMITTERS

Everything begins with the genes and their interactions with each other and their environment, but how does that translate into the behaviors and emotions of bipolar disorder?

In our brains, we have two kinds of cells: neurons, which transmit information throughout the brain and between the brain and body; and glial cells, which provide nutrients and other chemicals to the neurons, repair the brain if it's injured, and help defend the brain against infection. Our brains also include specialized proteins (hormones, enzymes, and neurotransmitters, among others) and chemicals, including calcium ions.

The neurons are the cells that send the messages telling our lungs to breathe and our hearts to pump. They receive and interpret data that tells us "That's Mom's face" and "My friend is happy to see me." They generate the signals that enable us to walk or run. They receive the signals that warn us that we're off-balance or about to step in a mud puddle, and they send messages out again so we can take corrective action.

And neurons send the signals that we express as behavior and emotion.

The messages that travel from neuron to neuron are electrochemical signals. Proteins called *neurotransmitters* trigger an electrical impulse in the neuron. The triggered neuron then releases its own neurotransmitters to trigger or suppress an electrical impulse in the next neuron down the line.

To understand how this works in our brain, let's begin with just two neurons. Neuron no. 1 has received a message, which it transmits to neuron no. 2 (Figure 1).

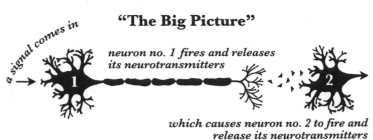

*Figure 1*

Now let's break the big picture down into smaller steps so we can see what's happening—and what can go wrong.

Each neuron has a cell body. Inside the body are vesicles—little sacks—packed with neurotransmitter molecules. Extending out from the body of the cell are branched segments called *dendrites* and one longer projection called an *axon* (Figure 2).

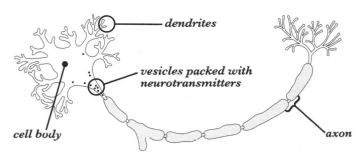

*Figure 2*

Inside the tip of each dendrite are receptors—special stations that neurotransmitters can enter, bind to, and release from. The dendrites extend like a dense forest of tiny filaments all around the neuron, waiting for neurotransmitters to drift by close enough to bind to a receptor.

Inside the axon, the vesicles filled with neurotransmitters are waiting at the cell membrane, like cargo trucks backed up to a wall of closed garage doors.

Receptors and neurotransmitters are specific for each

other; to bind, they have to fit together, like a key in a lock. Dopamine doesn't fit in a serotonin receptor; it needs a dopamine receptor to do its job.

When a neurotransmitter binds to a matching receptor, the receptor opens nearby channels that allow calcium ions to rush in or out of the neuron. The ions have a positive charge, so when the number of ions changes, the electrical charge or voltage near that receptor changes, too; it becomes more positive or more negative.

Which way the voltage changes depends on which channels the receptor activates, which in turn depends on the neurotransmitter. Some neurotransmitters are excitatory—they are sending a "Go!" message, telling the neuron to fire. Others are inhibitory, sending a "No!" message that prevents the neuron from firing.

One neurotransmitter in one receptor doesn't make a big enough change to make anything happen. It's the sum of all the receptor changes that determines whether or not the neuron will fire. It's like flipping a sticky switch. The "Go!" signals are pushing hard to flip the switch on. The "No!" signals are pulling hard to keep the switch off. When there are enough "Go!" signals to reach a critical point, called the *action potential,* the switch flips on and the electrical impulse travels through the neuron to its axon.

When the electrical signal hits the vesicles, they fuse with the membrane at the end of the axon and release their neurotransmitters. The cargo doors of the trucks roll up and the matching doors in the wall open. The cargo—the neurotransmitters—is pushed through the doors into the space on the other side of the wall.

The end of neuron no. 1's axon is very close to the dendrites of neuron no. 2. The tiny gap between the axon and its neighboring neuron is called the *synaptic cleft.* The neurotransmitters diffuse across this gap, ready to bind to the receptors on neuron no. 2's dendrites, and the whole process happens again in neuron no. 2.

The axon side of the synapse has receptors for neuro-transmitters, too. When a neurotransmitter binds to an axon-side receptor, it triggers a message to neuron no. 1 that says, "There's plenty of us out here, don't send any more." When neuron no. 1 receives enough of these messages, it stops releasing neurotransmitters until it receives a new signal from its dendrites causing it to fire again.

As the neurotransmitters bind and release from the receptors, other specialized proteins clear them out of the space, bringing them back into the neuron, where they are either recycled or deactivated (Figure 3).

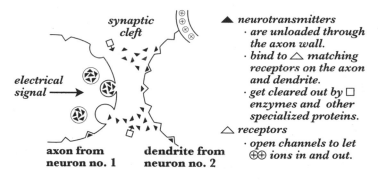

synaptic cleft

electrical signal ——▶

axon from neuron no. 1

dendrite from neuron no. 2

▲ *neurotransmitters*
· *are unloaded through the axon wall.*
· *bind to △ matching receptors on the axon and dendrite.*
· *get cleared out by □ enzymes and other specialized proteins.*
△ *receptors*
· *open channels to let ⊕⊕ ions in and out.*

*Figure 3*

There are several things that can happen to a neurotransmitter molecule after neuron no. 1 releases it through the axon.

- It can connect to a matching receptor on one of neuron no. 2's dendrites.

- If all the receptors are in use, it can drift around in the synaptic cleft until a receptor opens up, then bind to that receptor.

- It can bind to a receptor, release from the receptor, and bind to it or another matching receptor again.

- It can bind to a receptor on neuron no. 1, sending a "that's enough" signal.

- Enzymes and other special proteins can deactivate it in the synaptic cleft or carry it back into neuron no. 1, where it can be recycled or deactivated.

Even in this simple two-neuron example, there are plenty of things that can go wrong.

Neuron no. 1 might be making or releasing too much or too little of a particular neurotransmitter. It might be making a mistake when it manufactures the neurotransmitter, so it doesn't fit properly into the receptors on neuron no. 2 or can't disconnect from the receptor once it's bound. Neuron no. 1 might be reabsorbing its neurotransmitters too soon or be shutting down too early or continuing to release neurotransmitters despite repeated "that's enough" messages.

On neuron no. 2's side of the synapse, the receptors that it has manufactured might be defective, affecting their ability to bind, release, and respond to the neurotransmitters. There might be too many, not enough, or the wrong proportions of the ions flowing in and out of the channels, so neuron no. 2's voltage doesn't change as it should.

In the synaptic cleft between the two neurons, there might be an overabundance of the proteins that deactivate the neurotransmitters, so not enough of them reach the dendrites. Or the opposite might be true: not enough deactivation proteins, resulting in more neurotransmitters connecting with the dendrites for a longer time.

Neurons in our brains and bodies form vast, complicated networks. Some neurons communicate the way the two neurons in our example do. Other neurons send their signals to cells in muscles or glands. The process is still basically the same: When triggered, the neuron releases its neurotransmitters into the synaptic cleft, but instead of binding to receptors on another neuron, they bind to receptors on the cell of the muscle or gland. How the receiving cell responds depends on what kind of cell it is and—you guessed it—what neurotransmitter is involved. If enough motor neurons tell enough muscle cells in your big toe to twitch, your big toe twitches.

Neurons that send their signals to gland cells are connecting with our body's other major communication system. Gland cells—pituitary gland, hypothalamus, and other glands in the brain, and adrenal and other glands in our bodies—manufacture and release hormones.

When a hormone binds to a matching receptor on a cell, the receptor sends a signal that activates a small number of genes inside that cell. It turns those genes "on" so the cell can manufacture the proteins encoded by the genes. These proteins might turn on additional genes, which make other proteins. And, when enough genes in enough cells are producing enough proteins, they cause a result.

Here's an example of what this might look like on a bigger scale.

A collection of light and color—"visual data"—comes in through your eyes. The neurons in your optic nerve carry the data to the part of your brain that translates the data into something it can identify. "It's a lion," your brain says.

If you're alone on the African veld and the lion is running toward you, your neurons send signals to the cells involved in your fight-or-flight response, including the cells of your pituitary gland and adrenal glands. These glands release hormones (cortisol, adrenaline, and others) which communicate with other cells that need to supply the extra blood, oxygen, strength, and energy you'll need to escape the lion.

If, on the other hand, the lion is napping in the sun in the big cat compound at the zoo, your brain still says, "It's a lion," but it activates different neural pathways. You might feel awe or amusement or curiosity instead of fear. Instead of running or preparing to fight, you might stroll past the exhibit or stop long enough to read the sign describing lion habitat.

In both cases, the neurons of your optic nerve brought the

data into your brain's neural network. From there, signals traveled between neurons, gland cells, and muscle cells—but the end result, your emotions and behavior, were different, because the pathways the signals traveled within that network were different.

The different pathways are possible because different neurotransmitters and hormones are released along the way, causing some neurons to fire while suppressing others. The released hormones change how sensitive the receptors are, which changes how easy it is for an incoming signal to trigger the neuron. And at every step, the system provides feedback to itself—release more, that's plenty, fire again.

What happens if the brain makes a mistake? In the case of our lion, if the brain accurately recognizes "lion" but doesn't recognize "looks ready to attack me," it won't send the signal that activates your fight-or-flight system, and you'll be lion lunch.

At the zoo, if your brain recognizes "lion" but interprets what it sees as being dangerous, it ramps up the fight-or-flight system. You'll feel afraid or aggressive, ready to run or defend yourself. (This is part of what happens if you have a phobia of lions.)

There's another way the brain can make a mistake; it can misinterpret the lion itself. It interprets the data as "house cat" instead of lion and sends signals that tell you to pet the nice kitty. Or it interprets "house cat" as "attacking lion," and you confront ten pounds of confused tabby with an upturned chair.

In fact, we think something like this may explain some of the symptoms we see in bipolar.

In one study, researchers used pictures of human faces expressing different emotions. The face on one card was happy; the face on another sad or fearful. Some faces were neutral, that is, they did not show any emotion. The researchers showed the pictures to children and teens and asked them to identify the emotion on each card. The kids with bipolar often misinterpreted the neutral faces as showing hostility.

If you think the people around you are hostile, you'll react differently to them than if you think they're loving and friendly. Such misinterpretations may be part of the reason that kids with bipolar get angry, defensive, and suspicious and have a tough time in social situations; their brains are seeing a threat or rejection.

We don't know all the details of the pathways the signals travel. We do know that of the dozens of neurotransmitters that have been identified, several are certainly involved in mood disorders, because medications that change the levels of these neurotransmitters also change mood and behavior. The ones that seem especially important in bipolar are the mono-amines, which include serotonin, dopamine, and norepineph-rine; GABA (gamma-aminobutyric acid); and glutamate.

Figuring out what a drug does to change the level of a neurotransmitter also provides clues as to what might be mal-functioning in the neurons. For example, Risperdal (risperi-done), one of the medications used to treat bipolar, blocks dopamine receptors on the dendrite side of the synaptic cleft (it's a *dopamine antagonist*). Fewer open receptors means fewer dopamine molecules can bind, and the neuron won't fire as often as it would if Risperdal molecules weren't occupying some of the receptors. Risperdal's action decreases the amount of dopamine that can get to the next neuron.

The antidepressant Prozac is a *selective serotonin reuptake in-hibitor* (SSRI); it works on the axon side of the synapse, block-ing the receptors that take the serotonin back into the neuron for recycling and deactivation. Prozac's action increases the amount of time serotonin molecules spend in the synaptic cleft, which gives them more time to bind to their matching receptors on the other side of the synapse. It's similar to the effect we'd get if neuron no. 1 produced and released more serotonin.

Risperdal helps a lot of kids who have bipolar, and SSRIs trigger mania in some kids. Does that mean mania is caused by too much dopamine or too much serotonin?

Unfortunately, it isn't that simple. It probably isn't the level of one neurotransmitter that causes the problem, but the relative amounts of several. In addition, where the affected neurons are—which pathway in the network has the altered number of receptors or skewed ratio of neurotransmitters—makes a difference. Not enough dopamine in one area of the brain results in Parkinson's disease, a movement disorder. Not enough in another area affects thinking and memory. Combine the lower dopamine level with a higher or lower level of serotonin—in the same or different areas—and you'll get a different result.

There's another challenge in identifying which changes in neurotransmitters cause bipolar disorder. We don't always know whether the change we're observing caused the bipolar symptoms or whether something else caused the symptoms and, because of the feedback that happens through the system, the neurotransmitters changed as a result. In other words, did the change cause bipolar, or did bipolar cause the change?

For example, several studies demonstrated an increase in the number of one type of serotonin receptor in people who had depression. Did the increase in receptors cause their depression? Or did the cells make more receptors in response to too-little serotonin in the synaptic cleft? Or is the association between more receptors coincidental, unrelated to the depression? Other studies found a *decreased* number of a different serotonin receptor, especially in depressed people who had bipolar. Cause? Side effect? Coincidence?

These and other studies tell us that serotonin, dopamine, and other neurotransmitters are involved in causing the symptoms of bipolar, but they don't tell us how exactly they're involved.

## BRAIN STRUCTURE

Early in brain research, doctors and scientists recognized that certain brain injuries resulted in specific changes. Depending on what area of the brain was damaged, the patient might be unable to speak, recognize family members, or remember things. Some patients' entire personalities changed, from previously cheerful and even-tempered to suspicious and quick to anger (or vice versa). This supported the idea that the brain wasn't one homogeneous mass, but was organized into regions that were responsible for different functions. Some areas were concerned with thinking and conscious decision-making, others with emotions or movement.

As research has continued, our understanding of how the brain is organized is dovetailing with our understanding of how cell communication (neurotransmitters, hormones, and the genes that control them) works, providing a better picture of what is happening in the brain.

In other organs, each cell of the organ is essentially identical to all the other cells of that organ: One liver cell is pretty much like another. How those organ cells interact and what they do for the body are basically the same all the time.

Unlike other organs, the individual cells in our brains differ from each other. There are different types of cells, different shapes, and differences in the way each cell's machinery works and what job it does. There are literally trillions of possible connections and interactions possible between these cells. On top of these complex interactions among the genes, proteins, cells, and circuits of cells, there are interactions between the brain, the person, and the person's experiences. Our brains are changing all the time in response to the world around us.

Signals flow throughout this system like traffic in a big city. Without organization—if all the streets were narrow alleys and there weren't any stop signs or traffic lights—you'd have one giant traffic jam. Signals couldn't get to where they needed to be quickly enough, or they'd get snarled with other signals and never arrive at all.

The primary traffic control center is your *prefrontal cortex.* It's the front third of your brain, located underneath your forehead. The prefrontal cortex sends out the signals that tell you where to focus your attention. It keeps an eye on everything, guiding and directing your behavior in response to the information it receives. It enables you to think things through, manage your time, plan, organize, and control your impulses. An area of the prefrontal cortex called the *dorsolateral prefrontal cortex* (DLPC) helps you pay attention and is involved with your working memory (your short-term memory, where your brain stores information temporarily).

The prefrontal cortex also translates the signals it receives from your limbic system into recognizable sensations—the emotions you can name: fear, love, hate, and other feelings.

The *limbic system,* located deep in the center of your brain, is Grand Central Station for sensory information.

Data from our senses—sight, hearing, and so on—don't show up willy-nilly in our brains. The raw data from a particular sense—for example, vision data (light and color)—are received by areas in the brain specifically organized for that type of data.

Individual bits of data aren't information. We need to understand what all those bits of data mean. The limbic system receives data from the specialized areas of the brain and integrates, organizes, and interprets the data. As it does so, it provides emotional meaning to the information.

The limbic system is responsible for mood control. Its actions affect your sleep, appetite, sexual desire, and ability to bond. Its messages and processes control your fight-or-flight response. It stores memories that have strong emotional charges, too.

Problems within the limbic system are likely to cause problems elsewhere. Your prefrontal cortex makes decisions based on the information the limbic system sends to it. If the limbic system misinterprets the data, the prefrontal cortex will be making decisions based on bad information.

The limbic system includes several structures. Problems in any of them will affect emotions and behavior.

The *hippocampus* is involved in memory, learning, and spatial navigation (if you don't remember where you've been or how to get to where you're going, blame your hippocampus).

The *thalamus* is a relay station for incoming sensory data. It also regulates the level of awareness and activity—how awake you feel.

The *hypothalamus* links the nervous system to the endocrine system via the pituitary gland. It also controls body temperature, hunger, thirst, and circadian cycles.

The *amygdala* is involved in the processing and memory of emotional reactions and contributes to how strongly you react to a situation.

The *cingulate gyrus* enables us to shift from one thought or behavior to another, so we can see options and manage change and transitions. An overactive cingulate gyrus has been associated with getting stuck in thought loops and repetitive behavior (obsessive worries and compulsive behavior, for example).

The *temporal lobes* are involved in memory, understanding language, facial recognition, and anger control. Damage to the left temporal lobe has been associated with temper flare-ups, rapid mood shifts, and memory and learning problems.

The *basal ganglia* are large structures deep in the brain that work with the limbic system. They integrate thoughts, emotions, and movement—when you jump for joy, it's thanks to your basal ganglia. They're also involved in our feelings of motivation, pleasure, and ecstasy. Overactive basal ganglia have been associated with anxiety, panic, and fearfulness; underactive basal ganglia with problems in concentration and fine motor control.

Another area of the brain that we suspect is important in bipolar disorder is the *anterior cingulate cortex* (ACC). It's the front part of the cingulate cortex, which wraps around the bundle of nerve fibers that relay signals between the right and left side of your brain.

It is clear that the limbic system is involved in bipolar disorder. The DLPC and ACC systems probably are too; damage to the DLPC can result in impaired short-term memory and difficulty in inhibiting unacceptable or unwanted behavior. And the ACC seems to be involved in reward anticipation, decision-making, empathy, and emotions—all functions that are affected by bipolar disorder.

It's possible that some of the differences we see in the type and severity of symptoms may be related to specific structures within these systems. We don't yet know exactly what causes a system to malfunction or fail, but with newer technologies, we are beginning to identify what happens when different areas are affected.

## BRAIN IMAGING

If you break your arm, you get an X-ray that shows exactly where and how it's broken.

But what if your brain is broken?

Until recently, there was no way to directly examine the structure of a brain without surgery to "look under the hood." There was no way at all to identify function—which areas of the brain are active at any given time.

Brain imaging technologies are changing that. Newer technologies including magnetic resonance imaging (MRI), functional MRI (fMRI), positron-emission tomography (PET scans), computed tomography (CT scans), and spectroscopy are generating pictures of the "brain at work." Researchers are using brain imaging to explore how our brains function and what differences there are between healthy people and those who have mental illness, including bipolar.

We've learned a lot about brain function, but we are still a long way from understanding everything. It's tempting to look at a brain scan and say, "Ah! There's the problem, clear as a picture"—but right now, we don't have the data we need to diagnose a mental illness solely on the basis of a brain scan. As Jay Giedd, MD, chief of brain imaging in the child psychiatry branch of the National Institute of Mental Health, says, "Brain imaging in children is all about group averages—we are not good at determining the usefulness of individual brain scans yet."

Scans are a valuable tool for identifying physical problems in the brain—things like head trauma or a tumor. Scans may help some patients accept that their bipolar is truly a physical illness, which may in turn alleviate shame or denial they feel and reinforce the need for ongoing treatment.

Scanning technology continues to improve, and the database of scans continues to grow. Down the road, it's likely that scans will be combined with new knowledge about genetics and cell communication to pinpoint specific risk factors or problems.

We suspect in both children and adults that some combination of genetic vulnerability and environmental circumstance makes the stress-response system more sensitive, probably during early development. Later on, exposure to another stressor might trigger the illness in someone whose protective genetics—the high cards in their hand—aren't enough to compensate for the genetic vulnerability. It's likely that specific neurological systems are involved at different times of development.

A child's environment, both before and after birth, has a tremendous impact on brain development and subsequent behavior—but that doesn't mean you have to be a "perfect parent" or provide a "perfect environment" (which is good, because there isn't such a thing). Studies of different care-giving environments suggest that extreme environments such as severe abuse and neglect do affect brain survival and development as well as how the brain reacts to stress. But in cases that aren't extreme, researchers have found that kids' brains interact with their environment so that their brains are optimized for that environment. How you understand and behave in the world depends a lot on the type of world you're in.

The ability of our brain to let the environment influence the brain's neural circuitry is called *plasticity* or *malleability*. It's what allows the brain to continually adapt to its environment, which is an important part of learning and resilience. Experience changes the brain—learning has a physical effect— and these changes are mediated by the same signals and the same pathways in the brain that are affected by the medications we use to treat bipolar. The pathways are dependent on the individual's genotype—and we're back to where we started, working to identify what genetic vulnerabilities are involved, what protective elements (genetic and environmental) will help, and how it all works in the developing brain.

For someone close to a child or teen with bipolar, it can be frustrating to not know a specific cause. It may help to remember that it's only been since the 1990s that the medical and research community began to accept that children can have mood disorders. Now that we're starting to get a better idea of what to look for, research is pushing ahead to uncover causes, how the illness progresses, and how to treat and prevent it.

# Chapter 5

# SOUND BARRIER

## HOW TO TALK SO YOUR
## DOCTOR WILL HEAR

- "My kid has wicked bad temper tantrums."

- "My daughter sneaks out at night to party with her friends."

- "I suspect my teen is smoking pot, maybe getting into more serious drugs, too."

- "My son doesn't sleep; he puts up a major fuss at bedtime."

- "That child is crabby, crabby, crabby."

- "I worry because she seems so blue."

Practically every parent has said or thought at least one of these statements. Clinicians are used to hearing them, too.

But how blue is "blue"?

Teens are famous for adolescent moodiness and outrageous behavior. When is it ordinary rebellion and angst? When is it something more serious?

"My son puts up a fuss at bedtime" could mean anything from "He's tired and needs help getting into his pajamas" to "He throws furniture and screams so loudly the neighbors complain" or "He hasn't slept for four days—literally."

How do you help your child's doctor understand that you're not talking about behaviors or moods that are run-of-the-mill complaints? That this isn't just a phase or a rough patch or a short-term reaction to something new or temporary in your child's life? That just because your child is well behaved at this precise instant in the doctor's office does not mean you are exaggerating or overprotective?

During today's typical fifteen-minute doctor appointments, your clinician relies on you—your instincts as a parent and your observations of your child—to provide the information that says, "Pay attention: Something is wrong here."

For your clinician to understand and evaluate what's going on, she needs to know:

- what behaviors (or symptoms) worry you the most;

- how often the behaviors occur;

- how long the behaviors last; and

- how severe the behaviors are.

You need two things to get this information across:

1. A way to quickly and easily track your child's symptoms and behaviors. You and the clinician can use your records to gauge the frequency and severity of different symptoms and to identify trends and trouble spots.

2. Effective communication. By using specific language and concrete examples, you'll be able to convey the seriousness of your child's symptoms.

You'll use both of these techniques at the beginning, when you're trying to figure out what's causing your child's difficulties, and later, during treatment, to figure out what's working and what isn't.

Let's begin with two types of behavior that can be especially difficult to describe, severe "tantrums" and irritability.

## A RAGE STORM IS NOT A TANTRUM

Blowup. Meltdown. Eruption. Explosion.

Parents struggle to describe their child's intense, often frightening, sometimes dangerous, fury. These episodes can include screaming, profanity, and threats. They can be violent, with hitting, kicking, biting, and spitting. They can come out of nowhere or be triggered by things that seem trivial. They can be short and frequent or literally last for hours.

They are not temper tantrums.

They are manic explosions—an important symptom and challenging problem. We call them *rage storms*. Their character and quality are very different from typical childhood temper tantrums.

Most clinicians who hear the phrase "temper tantrum" automatically think, "Normal, ordinary childhood behavior"—and assume the parent is overreacting.

When you talk to your clinician, be clear that you are describing episodes that are abnormal: more intense, longer, more frequent, out of proportion to the trigger. Use phrases like "worse than anything I've seen in other children her age," combined with specific details about your child's rage storms (how long they last, how often they happen, and what kinds of behavior they include) to help your clinician understand that what your child is experiencing is far more severe than a tantrum.

## IRRITABILITY:
## AN OLD SYMPTOM, OFTEN IGNORED

One of the debates surrounding pediatric bipolar disorder concerns irritability, especially as a symptom of mania.

Early researchers studying bipolar in young children focused their attention on children whose manic symptoms were primarily or entirely euphoric, leading some clinicians to believe that a child must show signs of euphoria—over-the-top giddy, goofy, silly behavior—in order to have bipolar disorder. Irritability, they believe, isn't really a symptom of bipolar.

Others feel that practically everybody has irritability—it's so common that it can't be used to distinguish bipolar disorder from anything else—so they dismiss it as a symptom.

But irritability is a bona fide symptom—and not a new one. The DSM-IV criteria for mania, hypomania, and depression all include irritability as a possible symptom. The problem isn't whether or not irritability is a symptom—it is—but how we define it.

What do we mean by *irritable*?

Irritability, like the other symptoms of bipolar and the plus disorders, varies in severity.

There's low-level irritability: the common, everyday sensation we might feel when we're stuck in traffic or when a coworker interrupts us at an inconvenient time. Some days these little annoyances don't bother us; other days are "bad hair days" or "got up on the wrong side of the bed" days. We're more irritable, more likely to feel and act grumpy.

A step higher on the scale is the irritability that results from struggling with weak or trouble spots. For example, children (and adults) with ADHD often have a lower tolerance for frustration, and they have to work harder in certain areas to achieve the same results as someone who doesn't have ADHD. Frustration plus harder-than-it-should-be work leads to more intense irritation—bigger and longer scenes (grouchiness, refusing to do the work, angry outbursts), especially associated with the weak area.

Next is the irritability of depression. It ranges in severity, too, but it's a different "flavor" from the frustrated-with-the-trouble-spot irritation of ADHD and the irritability of mania. Children whose irritability stems from depression are more whiny, difficult to please, and joyless. Their irritability doesn't center on a particular task or weak area; it's more "all-around." They can be snippy, snappy, grouchy, and nasty.

The irritability of mania is at the top of the severity scale. Kids with manic irritability can be nasty, demanding, and vicious, with explosive, violent, and dangerous rage storms. Although there's a range of severity within manic irritability, most children with bipolar disorder will have significant, severe irritability that causes problems in their day-to-day life. In children, manic irritability is more common (and usually causes more problems) than euphoria.

You may not think of your child's rage storms, nonstop demands, and vicious name-calling as "irritability," but in terms of bipolar disorder, they are.

Your clinician may not think of "irritability" as a hallmark symptom, but it is.

Part of the problem is vocabulary: "Irritability" sounds like something that's a little bothersome, not something that's serious enough to disrupt lives and wreak havoc.

If you're having difficulty identifying irritability or convincing your clinician that it's a problem worth paying attention to, change your vocabulary. Instead of saying, "My daughter is extremely irritable all the time," try (for example), "My daughter is belligerent, caustic, mean, and wrathful most of the time, and she explodes in rages at least twice a day. Her bad mood and rages are much worse than those of other children her age." Looking for more ways to describe irritable? See "125 Ways to Be Irritable."

## 125 WAYS TO BE IRRITABLE

abrasive
acerbic
acrimonious
agitated
aggravated (and
    aggravating)
agonized
angry
anguished
bad-tempered
bearish
belligerent
bites your head off
bitter
blows his/her
    stack
boils over
bristling
burning
caustic
chafing
churlish
cranky
cross
defiant
despairing
discomposed
disgruntled
distressed
edgy
enraged
erupting

explosive
exposed nerve
fault-finder
fidgety
fit to be tied
flies into a rage
flies off the handle
flips out
foaming at the
    mouth
fractious
frantic
frenzied
fuming
furious
goes into a tailspin
goes through the
    roof
griping
grouchy
gruff
grumpy
having a fit
heckling
high-strung
hissy fit
hits the roof
hot under the collar
hotheaded
ill-at-ease
in a snit
incensed

indignant
infuriated
irascible
itching for a fight
livid
mad as a wet hen
mean
miserable
nettled
peeved, peevish
persecuted,
    persecuting
pestering
petulant
picked on, picking
    on
pissed off
plagued, plaguing
prickly
provoking
put-upon
querulous
rankled
ranting
raw
raw nerve
ready to explode
resentful
restless
riled, riled up
roiled and roiling
ruffled

| | | |
|---|---|---|
| savaging | tempestuous | unrestful |
| seeing red | tense | unsettled |
| seething | tetchy | upset |
| short fuse | tormented | vengeful |
| simmering | tortured | vexed |
| skittish | touchy | volcanic |
| smoldering | turbulent | whiny |
| snapping your nose | umbrageous | wild |
| off | unaccepting | wired |
| sour | uneasy | worked up |
| steamed | ungrateful | wrathful |
| sulky | unquiet | wretched |

## TRACKING SYMPTOMS

Symptoms of any illness vary from person to person and day to day. Look around your doctor's waiting room during cold and flu season. You'll notice plenty of runny noses. Some kids will be sitting quietly in Grandma's lap, while others will be howling or fidgeting. Some will cough or sneeze a little, some will cough long and hard.

It's pretty straightforward for the clinician to assess each child. We measure temperature to see who has a fever and who doesn't. We listen to hearts and lungs, peer into ears and throats. We ask where it hurts and swab the throat to test for bacteria.

It's more difficult to assess a mental illness such as bipolar disorder. There's no thermometer that measures how long and intense your child's temper tantrums are. Blood tests won't reveal how many holes your son has kicked in the walls. Lab work won't tell us if your daughter's distractibility is the kind that comes from ADHD, bipolar disorder, or the excitement of an upcoming holiday.

We need your observations, and the observations need

to be as specific and accurate as possible. Doctors and other clinicians think in terms of what they can observe. We need "just the facts, ma'am"—your specific observations about the moods, thinking, and behavior of your child. We need this information to figure out what's going on and what to do about it.

Parents are always searching for the answer to "why?" but *why* something happened isn't as important for diagnosis and immediate treatment as *what* happened. Was your daughter's reaction appropriate to whatever triggered the reaction? If she says, "I want to die" because she can't have a new toy, or if she trashes the house and breaks beloved items (yours or hers) because she lost a game, those are over-the-top, extreme reactions; they're out of proportion to their triggers. The *reason* she reacted (no toy, losing a game) isn't as important as the fact that her reaction was excessive.

When you track the frequency, intensity, and duration of your child's symptoms, you and your clinician will be able to look at the patterns of mood and behavior. These patterns help your clinician understand how your child's symptoms differ from those appropriate for children the same age.

Tracking your child's symptoms helps you keep your balance and perspective, too. Living day in and day out with your child's moods and disruptive behaviors can make you numb. Behaviors that are appalling and infuriating can seem ordinary if they happen all the time. Your struggle to simply get through the day becomes standard operating procedure for you and your family. Lousy days that aren't as horrible as awful days reinforce your hope that things aren't as bad as you fear. The occasional good day (or hour) adds to the cultural pressure to take the blame for your child's aberrant behavior. The combination of these factors often means that we wait too long to ask for help, we minimize the severity of the problem, and we doubt ourselves and our abilities as parents.

Track your child's symptoms. If you find yourself thinking things like, "Oh, I guess it really isn't that bad," or,

"Everybody's kids go through rough patches," or, "I'm the world's worst parent," check your records. Has your son's behavior nose-dived recently? Has your daughter's moodiness been off the charts for as long as you've had a chart? Records are a concrete reminder that you aren't imagining things. Your child really is struggling with something serious beyond his control.

You don't need to keep a record of everything your child feels, thinks, or does. Certainly if something strikes you as bizarre, over the top, or dangerous, you need to track it (and if it's dangerous—violent or suicidal behavior—get help immediately). For everything else, if it's enough of a problem that you're noticing it and worrying, it's worth tracking.

If a mood or behavior

- interferes with your child's ability to function (play, learn, enjoy friends and family, accomplish ordinary everyday tasks);

- affects the way your family functions (everybody's walking on eggshells, you feel like you're being held hostage, lots of strife and arguments centered around this particular child, disrupted family life); or

- raises your internal "red flag"

then it is severe enough to justify your attention. It isn't a "challenging behavior"; it's a symptom. These symptoms are the crucial clues that will lead to the help your child needs.

There are lots of ways to track your child's symptoms. We're illustrating three methods in this chapter, but any system that works for you is fine. Feel free to modify or combine these methods or create your own system. Remember: The goal is to provide a record of what's going on with the symptoms (mood, behavior) that worry you the most or cause a lot of difficulty for your child or family.

## USING A TRACKING CHART

Charts are one of the easiest ways to track behaviors and other symptoms.

You can use a ready-made chart like the MGH Pediatric Mania Symptom Checklist (Appendix C), but it probably makes more sense to create your own (from scratch or by modifying the MGH list).

Here's how it works.

Begin by deciding what symptoms you want to track. For many families, the most worrisome behaviors are the most destructive or disruptive ones—rage storms and other symptoms of manic irritability.

Your first list might look like this.

| | |
|---|---|
| awful tantrums (meltdowns, blowups) | |
| whiny, clingy | |
| cranky, grouchy | |
| hyper (bouncing around, won't pay attention, obnoxious) | |

Over time, you might add other behaviors or mood descriptions, perhaps because your child's symptoms changed or because you've identified a better (easier, more accurate, more helpful) symptom to follow. For example, your next list might look like this.

| | |
|---|---|
| rage storms | |
| whiny, babyish | |
| distractible | |
| restless energy, lots of movement | |
| annoying, obnoxious, defiant | |

Next, add the columns where you'll record your observations, including a column with space for notes.

Some parents record their observations daily (whenever they notice a symptom throughout the day or once a day), others every few days or once a week. We recommend that you record your information at least once a week, because otherwise, you're likely to forget what happened when.

Remember, you want to record information that will help your clinician quickly assess how troublesome your child's behaviors and other symptoms are. That information includes *frequency, duration,* and *severity.*

*Frequency* is simply the number of times you observe the behavior or symptom over a given time. It answers the questions "how often?" or "how many?"

If you're tracking symptoms daily, make a little tick mark as soon as you notice the behavior or jot down the total at the end of the day. If you're tracking weekly, record how often the behavior occurred during the week. You don't need to record the precise number of times; "many times per day, once a day, fewer than three days or more than four days per week" is enough detail to tell if this is a low- or high-frequency behavior.

You can also use codes to indicate frequency, which is especially helpful for symptoms that happen a lot: "1" if it happens fewer than five times, "2" for five to ten times, "3" for more than ten, for example. If you use a code, include a note on the chart indicating what each code means.

| SYMPTOMS | FREQUENCY | DURATION |
|---|---|---|
| *(behavior, mood, or other)* | *(how many, how often)* | *(how long it lasted)* |
| awful tantrums (meltdowns, blowups) | | |
| whiny, clingy | | |
| cranky, grouchy | | |
| hyper (bouncing around, won't pay attention, obnoxious) | | |

*Duration* is how long a particular symptom or behavior lasted. It's often considered part of severity—for example, a five-minute temper tantrum is usually less severe than a thirty-minute one.

*Severity* asks "how bad is it?" It's a measure of the type of behavior and its impact. Pounding a pillow is less severe than attacking siblings or destroying property; giggling that makes it hard to get homework done on time is less severe than laughing fits that disrupt everything and everyone. Making snide comments to her sister all morning is less severe than extreme irritability, foul language, and argumentativeness that make it impossible for her to be in the same room as anyone else.

It's hard to measure how long some symptoms last. When did her upbeat mood slide into giddy-goofy-silly? And it wasn't until after that two p.m. blowup that you realized she's been extra crabby for a while, too. In these cases, you'll rank

| SEVERITY | NOTES |
|----------|-------|
| *(how bad it was)* | *(important details, contributing factors, a word or two to jog your memory)* |
|  |  |
|  |  |
|  |  |
|  |  |

severity by how incapacitating the symptom is or by how much it interferes with her ability to function. You might not record anything at all for duration.

One of the simplest ways to record severity is to use a numbered ranking system. The higher the number, the more severe the episode. To make sure you're consistent, make a note on the chart indicating what qualifies as mild, moderate, severe, and extremely severe for the symptom you're tracking. Table 1 (page 104) shows a typical ranking we use for the severity of rage storms.

Your "Notes" column is a good place to record trends, triggers, and contributing factors ("missed afternoon meds"; "had sleepover at friend's house") or details that will help you remember particular episodes or situations ("bloodied brother's nose"). If you know that a reaction was completely out of proportion to its trigger—your son threw a severe tantrum because his sandwich had wheat instead of white bread, for

**TABLE 1**

| Code | Level | Includes These Behaviors |
|------|-------|--------------------------|
| + | mild | angry, yelling; no physical aggression |
| ++ | moderate | screaming, swearing, threatening, throwing things, hitting walls or breaking objects; no aggression toward another person |
| +++ | severe | loss of control; physical aggression that causes others to feel afraid |
| ++++ | extremely severe | police or emergency services intervention needed to keep child (and possibly others) safe |

example—make a note of it here. If your daughter becomes hyperactive, distractible, and over-the-top silly about the same time most days, note that.

You can keep a record of everything listed in the chart right from the start, but more likely, you'll begin by simply tracking a few major symptoms, like Jennifer in the following example.*

At first, Cameron's mom, Jennifer, thought he had a particularly bad case of the "terrible twos." Her friends sympathized, but as his tantrums got worse, they stopped inviting Cameron to play dates. Jennifer read everything she could

---

*The examples in this chapter draw from the experiences of many parents. The information in the examples is for illustration only and is not an actual record for a specific individual.

find on parenting toddlers, but none of the suggestions worked. The first few times she talked to the pediatrician about Cameron's tantrums, he acknowledged that kids this age are challenging, especially kids as bright and creative as Cameron. Jennifer's intuition told her that there was more to Cameron's behavior than that.

Like everyone, Cameron had good days and bad days. Bad days seemed like one continuous tantrum. Good days— well, good days had tantrums, too, Jennifer realized, just not as many.

She began to keep a daily chart of his tantrums. The first week, she recorded times and notes about specific behaviors. At the end of the first week, she streamlined her record-keeping and, at the end of the second week, she made a follow-up appointment with the pediatrician (see charts, pages 106–107).

One look at the chart told the pediatrician that Jennifer's intuition was right. The frequency and severity of Cameron's tantrums were well beyond the norm for toddlers. His outbursts were persistent severe rages, not the normal tantrums of childhood.

Jennifer tracked Cameron's tantrums because that behavior was the one she and everyone else noticed the most. It wasn't his only symptom—on Saturday, Week 1, she wrote, "grumpy and fussy all day"—but for Cameron, tracking temper tantrums was the place to start, and the place to begin communicating how different he was from other kids his age.

Jennifer began tracking other symptoms, which helped the pediatrician make a tentative diagnosis of pediatric bipolar disorder. He recommended that Cameron see an advanced practice psychiatric nurse who specialized in treating young children who had mood disorders. Since then, Jennifer has continued to use charts to track Cameron's symptoms. From these records, she and Cameron's treatment team are better able to understand what's going on with Cameron and his illness.

**JENNIFER'S CHART, WEEK 1**

| Monday | Tuesday | Wednesday | Thursday | Friday | Saturday | Sunday |
|---|---|---|---|---|---|---|
| 10 a.m. 1/2 hr. tantrum. fell asleep on floor 15 min. woke up screaming. more tantrum. 2-2:30 hitting. screaming. crying. 4:00 threw snack on floor (mad). 15 min. screaming 5-6. threw blocks at window | Bad day. head banging. kicking. screaming. ALL DAY | 1:00. 20 min. kicking. pounding on floor. OK rest of day | 8:30 10 min. tantrum 10:00. 20 min. 11:15. 5 min. 4:00 1/2 hour 9:00 half hour | 10:00. 1/2 hr. tantrum 1:30. LONG time—1 hour? | no tantrums! but grumpy and fussy all day | 10:00. 1/2 hr. hated breakfast. threw cereal bowl. kicking. etc. 1:00. 20 min. started in grocery store. hitting. kicking. screaming. more in car and at home |

# JENNIFER'S CHART, WEEK 2

| Monday | Tuesday | Wednesday | Thursday | Friday | Saturday | Sunday |
|---|---|---|---|---|---|---|
| ✓ 2 ++ | ✓ 3 ++ | ✓ ) +++ | ✓ ) + | ✓ 2 + | ✓ 3 +++ | ✓ ) + |
| ✓ 2 ++ | ✓ 3 +++ | ✓ 2 ++ | ✓ ) ++ | ✓ 3 +++ | ✓ 3 ++ | ✓ 2 ++ |
| ✓ 3 +++ | ✓ 3 ++ | ✓ 2 ++ | ✓ ) ++ | ✓ 2 +++ | | ✓ ) + |
| ✓ 2 ++ | | | ✓ ) +++ | | | |
| ✓ ) + | | | ✓ ) +++ | | | |
| | | | | | | |

✓ = new tantrum. 1 = less than 5 min.; 2 = 5–10 min.; 3 = longer than 10 min.
+crying, screaming; ++plus throwing toys, etc.; +++plus hitting, kicking (things or people)

USING A MEDICATION LOG

Some parents track the medications their child takes using the same chart they use to track symptoms. Others use a medication log. Using a log like this one provides a quick visual—you can see when meds changed, or what she was taking "back when." You don't need to record the information every day, since you usually try a particular course of medication for a while. Update it when you add a medication, change a dose, or discontinue a medication, or update it every three months. When you discontinue a medication, you can use the blank line that results to record a note about why that medication was dropped (e.g., weight gain, lethargy, made symptoms worse).

| Date | Name of Medications | | |
|---|---|---|---|
| In this column, record the date your child began taking a medication, began a different dosage, or stopped using a medication. | Record the name of the medication here. | Record the name of the medication here. | Record the name of the medication here. |
| | Record the dosage of the medication listed above here. | Record the dosage of the medication listed above here. | Record the dosage of the medication listed above here. |

## USING A DAILY PLANNER OR CALENDAR

Charts don't work for everyone. If you're the kind of person who's lost without a daily planner or calendar, you can use it to record your observations. Again, the purpose is not to track every detail, but to capture enough information for a clear picture of your child's symptoms over time.

Here's how Jennifer can track Cameron's temper tantrums and moods using a day planner.

| Monday | Monday | |
|---|---|---|
| | 8:00 a.m. | |
| | 9:00 | * |
| | 10:00 | T/+++ |
| Notes | 11:00 | |
| ɛvɛ.⁻ threw blocks at window | 12:00 | ↑ |
| | 1:00 | |
| | 2:00 | |
| | 3:00 | * |
| | 4:00 | |
| | 5:00 | T/+++ |
| | 6:00 | |

In this example, Jennifer writes "T" for "temper tantrum" next to the time the outburst began and +, ++, or +++ to indicate how severe the tantrum was. She also notes when Cameron's moods are pronounced—an up arrow for silly, goofy, giddy; a down arrow for blue or sad; and a star for irritable. She jots down brief details in the "Notes" section that might be useful.

Here's how the same information might look on a wall calendar. This approach has a little less detail because Jennifer isn't tracking when Cameron's moods shift. We can tell from her records that on Monday, his mood was either "irritable" or "up" enough to be noticed. She can also jot down the time she noticed a shift in mood or other details that help her remember what happened on that particular day.

| 10 | 11 | 12 | 13 | 14 | 15 | 16 |
|---|---|---|---|---|---|---|
| | T +++ <br> T +++ <br> ★↑★ <br> (blocks) | | | | | |

## USING A JOURNAL

Some parents record their observations in a daily journal. The advantage of a journal is that you're likely to include your own reflections and insights about the day's events, which may help you identify triggers, trends, and patterns. Journal entries can also put symptoms in context, so you have a better view of the big picture. The disadvantage of a journal is that sometimes it can be hard to find specific information when you need it.

There are as many ways to keep a journal as there are people writing them. Maybe you've been pouring heart and soul onto the pages of a diary since you were ten. Maybe your journal reads like the captain's log from *Star Trek* or a to-do list. You might write longhand or type into a file on your computer or personal blog. The method you use doesn't matter; what matters is that you can find the specific, relevant information you need, when you need it. Here's an example.

Angela* got off to a rough start this school year. Her favorite teacher retired, her best friend moved, and, as a fourth-grader, she spends mornings in one classroom and afternoons in another. With all the changes and upheaval, no one was surprised that she was having some difficulty. But eight weeks into the semester, when her mother, Sara, took her to see their family doctor, she was still having problems. Angela seemed sad and blue a lot of the time, though she did perk up in the evenings. Her grades were mostly Cs, even in the subjects she'd always enjoyed and done well in. Her teacher had mentioned that Angela seemed to worry a lot and was having trouble concentrating, too.

Angela's doctor prescribed Zoloft, an antidepressant used to treat depression and anxiety. About a week after she began taking the Zoloft, Angela started feeling crabby and irritable. Her irritability escalated, and when they returned for a follow-up appointment, the doctor thought the irritability was a side effect of the Zoloft. Perhaps a different antidepressant would be more effective.

Something about this "new" behavior niggled at the back of Sara's memory. Angela had always been a pretty good kid, but she did get prickly from time to time. Before trying another medication, Sara skimmed through her journal entries for the last few months. She realized that Angela's irritability had actually begun to increase in early summer. Angela's

*The examples in this chapter draw from the experiences of many parents. The information in the examples is for illustration only and is not an actual record for a specific individual.

energy level had been a lot higher in the evenings starting around the same time, too, Sara noted. At the time, she'd assumed it was because of long summer days, and she'd blamed Angela's crabbiness on not getting enough sleep.

When Sara told the doctor what she'd found, he agreed that something other than depression might be behind Angela's moodiness.

June 18—Talked with Mom on the phone this morning. She's volunteering at the library's summer reading program again, loves it but of course couldn't resist telling me how nice all the kids are, not one ever makes a nasty comment, not to her, not to another kid. She didn't say "unlike Angela," but I knew she was thinking it.

July 25—Whew, what a day. Angela passed her dolphin level at swim lessons, I swear she's half fish. We celebrated with pizza for supper, which she wanted and then refused to eat. Better after supper, though she bounced all over her room until midnight, then complained she couldn't sleep because of weird noises in her room. I finally had to sit there until she fell asleep. Good thing we still have that beanbag chair. I am SO tired.

August 5—...I cannot believe my own daughter would say such a thing. I told her she's grounded for a month, absolutely we will not go shopping, and of course Mom says I should have washed her mouth out with soap...

| | | |
|---|---|---|
| **"terrible"** | your cousin means her kid throws a hissy fit about once a month | you mean that your kid throws anything he can get his hands on— lamps, books, dishes, shoes, the dog—during daily meltdowns |
| **"explosive"** | your child's psychologist means behavior that includes shouting and lots of door slamming | you mean behavior that includes breaking things |
| **"no symptoms"** | your child's doctor thinks, "No problems" | you think, "We can't keep this up. We're walking on eggshells. Life revolves around this kid for the very practical reason that it's the only way to avoid all kinds of problems and disruptions" |
| **"it's not so bad"** | your neighbor means that her kid talks back to her every once in a while | you mean you've been coping so long with extreme problem behaviors that you're numb, exhausted, and have forgotten (if you ever knew) how other kids behave |

## BREAKING THE SOUND BARRIER:
## HOW TO GET YOUR MESSAGE ACROSS

Once you've gathered a record of the symptoms that worry you, it's time to meet with your child's clinician. Initially, your records will help identify whether your child's moods and behaviors are above and beyond those of most children of the same age. After your child is diagnosed (whether the diagnosis is bipolar disorder or something else), you'll continue to track symptoms so that you and your child's treatment team can see what's working and catch problems as early as possible.

When you meet with the clinician or other member of the treatment team, you're going to do two things: Bring a copy of your records (the tracking chart, a summary of your calendar notes, highlights from your journal, or other information you've kept along with any medical records, including dose, side effects, and response) to share with the doctor; and talk about your observations using *specific language* and *concrete examples*.

The typical comments we began this chapter with may be true, but they aren't specific or concrete. That's why it's hard for your doctor to know whether you're describing normal (even if it's unpleasant) behavior, a rough patch that will get better on its own, a parenting or situational problem, or a significant medical problem that needs immediate attention.

Specific language includes how often and how severe a symptom is. Concrete examples include brief descriptions of your observations.

Here are some examples, using those earlier, more general comments.

*General:* "My kid has wicked bad temper tantrums."

*Specific language:* "In the last week, my kid has thrown seventeen temper tantrums. Four of them lasted more than twenty minutes and all of them were triggered by something minor."

*Concrete example:* "Her tantrums are unlike anything I've

seen in other kids. They include hitting, kicking, screaming, and sometimes biting. Her first meltdown on Tuesday started when I told her she couldn't have ice cream for breakfast. She threw her cereal bowl at me and spent the next half hour on the kitchen floor, kicking, pounding, and screaming."

In this example, the parent has described behavior that is definitely more severe than we'd expect from any child, regardless of age. The three big clues are the frequency (seventeen tantrums in a week); the severity (they last a long time and include hitting, kicking, and biting); and big reactions to small triggers (a reasonable request—no ice cream—resulted in a major meltdown).

*Specific language:* "My kid throws a tantrum whenever I tell him he can't have something. He's always been a little defiant, but these temper tantrums are new. They last about five minutes or so, but they're fierce—he's loud, his face gets bright red, he kicks and tries to bite."

*Concrete example:* "Yesterday, he saw a commercial on TV for a new squirt gun. He wanted to go to the store right away and buy it. First no of the day, and first temper tantrum—it lasted only a couple of minutes, but fifteen minutes later, he asked again; second no, second tantrum. The whole day was like that, like a series of explosions one right after the other."

The tantrums described by this parent may not be quite as severe as those in the first example, but they are much more frequent. Their trigger—Mom saying, "No, you can't have that toy"—is small compared to the intensity of the tantrum. The concrete example also contains clues about other symptoms: The repeated asking for a toy may be an element of mania ("activities with bad outcomes," the "A" of DIGFAST), and the frequently occurring tantrums might be part of severe irritability, another indicator of mania.

*General:* "My daughter sneaks out at night to party with her friends."

*Specific language:* "My daughter routinely breaks curfew.

If we ground her, she waits until we're asleep and then sneaks out. She's done this occasionally before, but it's getting worse. Last week, she came home at three in the morning on a school night; Friday, she stayed out all night; and she tried to sneak out again on Saturday night. She brags that there's nothing we can do to stop her."

*Concrete example:* "On Wednesday, when we caught her climbing through her window in the wee hours, she couldn't stop giggling. She swore she wasn't drunk or stoned, but I'm not convinced. The 'friends' she hangs out with are older, not kids from her high school."

*General:* "I suspect my teen is smoking pot, maybe getting into more severe drugs, too."

*Specific language:* "He doesn't come home on time and refuses to tell us where he's been. His behavior the past week has ranged from over-the-top goofy (two evenings) to open defiance and verbal abuse (every day). He refuses to do chores and says he's done his homework when it's obvious he hasn't."

*Concrete example:* "His coach called and asked why he hadn't been to practice all week, the first we knew he'd skipped. When we confronted him, he said the coach was a jerk and he didn't need to go."

Again, the specific information paints a clearer picture of how severe the problem is. The combination of behaviors observed in both of these teens—defiance, rule-breaking, bragging, lying, extreme giddiness—tells us that something more than typical teen rebellion is going on.

*General:* "My son doesn't sleep; he puts up a major fuss at bedtime."

*Specific language:* "My son has always been a night owl, even when he was a baby. I noticed last summer that he got more wound up in the evenings, talking a lot, wanting to wrestle or climb on the furniture, so we moved his bedtime back.

When school started, he couldn't get to sleep at bedtime even though we got him up in time for school. Most nights, he's sleeping only four or five hours. He falls asleep more easily if one of us sits beside him in his room, but even then, he rarely falls asleep before eleven. Last week, he was awake past eleven on four nights and past midnight twice. It takes over an hour for him to wake up and get ready for school, but once he's up, he doesn't seem tired."

*Concrete example:* "Wednesday was typical. He was a chatterbox at supper, talking a mile a minute, mostly about school. Lots of joking, funny stuff, but we had to keep reminding him that some jokes aren't okay at the dinner table. After supper, he couldn't settle. He kept pacing from room to room, up and down the stairs, for about an hour. Quieted down a little when we did bedtime reading, but he was still wide awake. He finally fell asleep a little after eleven."

Some people, kids included, are more night owl than early morning lark, something this parent has already taken into account. As she's tracked her son's sleep problems, she's also noticed several other important symptoms (talkativeness, inappropriate jokes, hyperactivity) that surface consistently.

*General:* "That child is crabby, crabby, crabby."

*Specific language:* "She's crabby and irritable almost continuously. Her behavior toward her sister has been especially nasty this last week—vicious name-calling, wrecking toys. We're walking on eggshells all the time, trying to avoid setting her off."

*Concrete example:* "Tuesday was a 'Jekyll and Hyde' day. Everything seemed fine until about ten o'clock. Her mood slid downhill and by eleven, she'd tried to pick a fight with her sister four times and had ripped the heads off several dolls, including two of her own favorites. Nothing I tried made her feel any better. She was crabby and angry—nasty name-calling, arguing—or weepy and clingy, sometimes both, for the rest of the day."

*General:* "I worry because she seems so blue."

*Specific language:* "She's weepy and mopes around the house. She won't talk to her friends when they call, and she spends most evenings in her room. She seems 'prickly'— irritable, not just unhappy. Twice this week, she refused to go to school, saying she was too tired to do anything. When I tried to cajole her into going, she said it wouldn't matter because she was stupid, and everybody knew it."

*Concrete example:* "When I encourage her to join the rest of the family instead of hiding in her room, she either snaps at me and says to leave her alone or gets very weepy."

Tracking and describing your child's moods can be difficult. Words like crabby, irritable, angry, silly, happy, and sad mean different things to different people. Whenever possible, include specific behaviors that help clarify what you mean when you say "crabby."

Kids arc also likely to be "spinning stars," shifting rapidly between moods or feeling different moods at the same time. If your child's moods seem like a muddled mess and you're not sure what's going on, note what you see. That might be specific behaviors (nasty name-calling, clinginess, avoiding friends) or overall impressions (Jekyll and Hyde, walking on eggshells, prickly).

## SOME BARRIERS ARE BIGGER THAN OTHERS

Your child's symptoms may have erupted suddenly, like a surprise case of chicken pox. The change in mood or behavior was clear and definite.

Perhaps your child's symptoms developed gradually over time, wobbly moods and worrisome behaviors bothersome, then frustrating and aggravating, finally graduating to alarming.

Or perhaps your child arrived in the world already struggling with severe symptoms, symptoms that shifted and changed over time, making it hard to link them to the same cause.

Tracking your child's symptoms, whether you've been doing it for years or just since yesterday, is the starting point for evaluating your child's difficulties. If, despite your best efforts and the supporting evidence of the information you've recorded, your child's clinician doesn't take your concerns seriously, it's time to get a second opinion. It doesn't matter why you can't break through your doctor's sound barrier (there are lots of possible reasons); what matters is that you find a professional who will listen, discuss and explore your concerns, and help you and your child.

# TRACKING CHART

**Date (or day of the week)** _____

| TIME OF DAY | SYMPTOMS | FREQUENCY | DURATION | SEVERITY | NOTES |
|---|---|---|---|---|---|
| | *(behavior, mood, or other)* | *(how many, how often)* | *(how long it lasted)* | *(how bad it was)* | *(important details, contributing factors, a word or two to jog your memory)* |
| | | | | | |
| | | | | | |
| | | | | | |

Severity: 1=mild; 2=moderate; 3=severe; 4=extremely severe

Symptoms can be specific behaviors (for example, hitting), a cluster of behaviors (a rage storm might include screaming, name-calling, hitting, kicking, and more, depending on the severity), an emotion or attitude (goofy, giddy, silly, crabby, cranky, nasty, defiant), or a combination of these. For more ideas on specific symptoms to include, see Appendices B and C.

# TRACKING CHART

Week of _____

| TIME OF DAY | SYMPTOMS (behavior, mood, or other) | FREQUENCY (how many, how often) | DURATION (how long it lasted) | SEVERITY (how bad it was) | NOTES (important details, contributing factors, a word or two to jog your memory) |
|---|---|---|---|---|---|
| | | 1 2 3 4 | 1 2 3 4 | 1 2 3 4 | |
| | | | | | |
| | | | | | |
| | | | | | |

Frequency, per week: 1 = less than 3 days; 2 = 4 or more days; 3 = every day; 4 = many times every day
Duration, per week: 1 = fleeting (a few minutes or less); 2 = brief (up to 15 minutes); 3 = moderate (15 to 60 minutes); 4 = prolonged (hour or longer)
Severity, per week: 1 = mild; 2 = moderate; 3 = severe; 4 = extremely severe
Symptoms can be specific behaviors (for example, hitting), a cluster of behaviors (a rage storm might include screaming, name-calling, hitting, kicking, and more, depending on the severity), an emotion or attitude (goofy, giddy, silly, crabby, cranky, nasty, defiant), or a combination of these. For more ideas on specific symptoms to include, see Appendices B and C.

# Chapter 6

# HIDDEN ALLIES

## FINDING THE RIGHT PEOPLE FOR YOUR CHILD'S TREATMENT TEAM

Pediatric bipolar disorder is a complex and complicated illness. Kids grow and change rapidly; symptoms come and go and change form. The chaos bipolar leaves in its wake affects everyone in the child's world and puts tremendous stress on the family. Treatment is going to take more than a quick trip to your child's pediatrician—it's going to take an entire team.

Your child's treatment team will include people with different skills from different fields. We call these people "hidden allies" because it may take some searching on your part to find the right people.

The people on the team will probably change over time because your child's needs will change. For example, you'll need a psychiatrist or advanced practice nurse on your team. When your child is young, you need someone who works with young children. You may need to switch to a different doctor— one who specializes in teens or young adults—when your child is older.

Other team members might be family therapists, couples counselors, or social workers. You might need an advocate to help navigate health insurance policies or educational support programs. Your team might include a lawyer, a contact at the local emergency room, a liaison in the local police department, a support group, and your family doctor.

Finding the hidden allies who will help you and your child is a challenging task, and it can be intimidating. This chapter will guide you in your search. You'll learn what skills to look for, where to look, and what questions to ask. You'll know what to expect when you and your child meet a specialist for your first visit or evaluation. You'll understand how to match the problems and difficulties that arise from your child's illness with the talents and specialties of potential team members.

With these skills in place, you'll be ready to form a powerful treatment partnership.

## ALLIES FROM ALL QUARTERS

*Andrew's team includes an advanced practice psychiatric nurse (diagnosis five years ago, ongoing treatment), a neurologist (concerns about suspected problems with muscle tone, a muscle tic, and shuffling gait), an occupational therapist and speech therapist (for nonverbal learning disabilities), a support group, an educational advocate, and his parents.*

It takes a village to raise a child, so the saying goes. If your child has bipolar disorder, it takes a bigger village.

Caring for and raising a child who has bipolar requires a multidisciplinary approach: different professionals who specialize in different areas. Who you need on your team and when depends on what your child needs. The medications that help manage your son's extreme irritability and violent outbursts don't solve his problems with low self-esteem or learning disabilities. The therapy that improves your daughter's mood management skills won't, on its own, solve the bigger challenge of family isolation and disrupted relationships.

We've divided these specialists into four categories: medical, therapeutic, educational, and friends and family. Your team will include allies from all four.

## MEDICAL

There are two main groups of medical allies: those who focus on physical health, such as pediatricians and family physicians, and those who focus on mental health, psychiatrists and advanced practice psychiatric nurses, for example. Both groups include medical doctors, nurse practitioners, physician assistants, and other professionals with special training in medicine.

Both groups also have lots of different specialties within them. A specialist in one field may be familiar with other fields, but he won't have the same level of expertise in them as he has in his own. There are specialists within fields, too. Some of the medical allies who are likely to be on your team are listed below.

*Primary Care Provider (PCP).* This is who you take your child to for routine healthcare, from well-child checkups to worrisome fevers and more serious concerns. Your PCP can be a medical doctor, a nurse practitioner, or a physician assistant and probably specializes in pediatrics or family medicine.

*Psychiatrist.* A medical doctor with advanced education and training in diagnosing and treating mental illness. Psychiatrists can provide therapy and prescribe psychiatric medications.

*Advanced Practice Psychiatric Nurse.* An advanced practice nurse who specializes in mental health. Advanced practice nurses are registered nurses (RNs) who have advanced education in diagnosing and treating mental illness. Depending on their role, they may be called a clinical nurse specialist or a nurse practitioner. Like psychiatrists, advance practice nurses can provide therapy and prescribe psychiatric medications.

*Neurologist.* A medical doctor with advanced education and training in disorders of the nervous system, including the brain. Historically, neurology, with its focus on the physical structures of the brain and nervous system, and psychiatry, which emphasized the intangible "mind," were considered entirely separate disciplines. As research continues to show that illnesses once considered to be "neurological diseases" often have a mental illness component and illnesses once described as "mental illnesses" are the result of neurological problems, the two disciplines are overlapping more and more.

*Hospital Personnel,* including emergency medical personnel (emergency room doctors, nurses, staff; emergency medical technicians). Many—perhaps most—kids with bipolar disorder require hospitalization at some point during their illness. If you're in the midst of a crisis—a suicide attempt or severe manic episode—your child's route to the hospital may be through the emergency room. In other situations, your child may be admitted to the psychiatric ward of a hospital, a psychiatric hospital, or other residential care facility. All of these facilities have medical professionals with varying degrees of experience and expertise in bipolar and other mental illnesses. (Chapter 11 includes more information about hospitalization.)

*Other medical specialists.* A child with bipolar isn't immune to other ailments. In addition to the medical challenges that might confront any child, some kids with bipolar may develop an increased risk for diabetes. Changing medications may solve the problem, but sometimes you may need to add an *endocrinologist* to the treatment team. Endocrinologists specialize in diabetes and other disorders of the pancreas, reproductive organs, and pituitary, adrenal, and thyroid glands, which make up the endocrine system.

An *insurance advocate* is another useful team member. Insurance advocates may be independent, employed by your health insurance company, or employed by your employer. They help you identify what services are covered under your health insurance policy and help resolve problems regarding payments and other issues. Although they generally don't have advanced medical training like the other allies in this category, their skill at navigating the often-confusing insurance terrain can be invaluable. If your insurance company denies a claim or coverage, you can appeal the decision. Appeals usually begin with asking your clinician to write a note to the insurance company explaining why the services are in the best interest of your child.

*Derick is thirteen; he's been seeing mental health specialists since he was seven. He and his mom, RaeAnn, have come to the clinic to participate in one of our research studies.*

*RaeAnn found out about the study online and decided to apply, even though it meant flying to Boston from their home in New Mexico and staying in a hotel for several days. Like many of our study participants, she wants to learn more about treatment and prognosis. RaeAnn also hopes to get a clearer diagnosis. Their doctor back home agrees that Derick is very ill with mood disorders, but Derick's symptoms don't fit with what he knows about bipolar.*

*During our time together, we discuss Derick's symptoms, what meds he's taking, and how he's responded to other medications in the past.*

*It's clear that mania is causing many of Derick's symptoms. Extreme irritability, anger, defiance, and oppositional behavior have been problems. About a year ago, the anger became much worse. RaeAnn thought it might be a meds problem—they'd tried many different meds and nothing seemed quite right—so they discontinued everything. Derick's behavior and mood nose-dived. He spent the summer as an outpatient in a psychiatric hospital, then was hospitalized for a while. His behavior included physical aggression, especially toward his siblings, and frequent rages with shouting and screaming that lasted more than half an hour. Holding him seemed to make it worse.*

*Derick is also funny and entertaining, but sometimes he's*

*provocative and his "jokes" are over the top or inappropriate. He can be "silly-goofy-giddy" and talkative, but RaeAnn says his speech isn't speedy or pressured. "It's more like he's impatient, worried that he's going to forget what he wants to say," she explains. This leads to a discussion of Derick's fidgetiness and distractibility.*

*Derick also has a lot of anxiety. When RaeAnn hears that half of the kids who have bipolar also have an anxiety disorder and that learning disabilities are surprisingly common, she nods her head emphatically. She's suspected that Derick might have a learning disability that's been missed because all the attention has been on the mood disorder.*

*By the time RaeAnn and Derick head home, they have confirmation of Derick's bipolar diagnosis plus new diagnoses of anxiety disorder and ADHD; a plan to have Derick tested for learning disabilities; and recommendations for adjusting Derick's meds. At RaeAnn's request, we'll also send a copy of our recommendations to their doctor and be available to answer questions he may have.*

*We've been on Derick's treatment team for a little over half a day; that was plenty to help Derick and his mom move along in his treatments.*

## THERAPEUTIC

Therapeutic allies include therapists, counselors, and psychologists. These allies have advanced degrees—a master's degree in social work or a doctorate in clinical psychology, for example—but not medical or nursing degrees. Unlike psychiatric professionals, therapeutic allies don't prescribe medications or other medical treatments, but, like psychiatrists, they often specialize in a particular age group or illness. Most also specialize in a particular type of therapy; family therapy and cognitive behavioral therapy are two common types used to help families affected by bipolar. (Chapter 8 has more information on specific types of therapies.)

Jonathon's team includes a psychiatrist, an endocrinologist, a nutritionist, his mom and stepdad, and his camp counselor at a special summer camp program.

## EDUCATIONAL

Kids with bipolar and bipolar plus need support and accommodations to succeed in school. These services are usually provided through your school district's special education department. An independent educational advocate can help you sort through the laws governing special ed as well as the programs and options that are appropriate for your child.

You're not required to use an advocate to get educational support for your son or daughter; in fact, many parents serve as their child's educational advocate on their own. Others consult an advocate only when they need extra help, fresh ideas, new strategies, or assistance in resolving problems.

Within the school system itself, educational allies include special ed teachers, school guidance counselors, and other school professionals and staff. (Chapter 9 has more information on how to obtain supports and services that will help your child succeed in school.)

*I searched out educational professionals, people who were supposed to know about kids. I read lots, and I sought out other kinds of professionals. Honestly, I wanted someone to say, "Yes, you are a bad parent," because that's something I could fix! One therapist kept pushing the behavioral part, but I knew there was a missing link. My son's behavior wasn't the only piece.*

*Each day started out with a huge tantrum. My husband left us and the therapist said that's what caused the problems, even though the tantrums had been going on for years before that. People told me it was temperament, some kids are harder than others. Our regular doctor said my son was just "all boy" and wouldn't refer us to the psychiatric center, and the center wouldn't see us without our pediatrician's referral.*

*When my son was in the sixth grade, a good friend whose kids have ADHD recommended a doctor who specialized in autism. My son was in major crisis, extremely explosive, flipping coins nonstop in his room, hearing voices, telling me that God was talking to him, really paranoid. The autism specialist was good at hand-holding. He was the first person outside of a few wonderful teachers who really believed that my son's behavior was a symptom. He tried one of the new medications, but it didn't work. Then my son went into a manic state that I'd never seen before. He was completely uninhibited, he'd do and say anything, anywhere. He continually made sexually laced comments. I was mortified, even though I knew he didn't know what he was doing. We had two big meetings at the school; they treated it like the emergency it was. We tried a lot of things but it was too late. His behavior spiraled down fast, and he couldn't be in school. The school found a residential program and got him into it twenty-four hours later.*

*Somewhere in all this, somebody mentioned a support group. It was facilitated by a psychiatric nursing specialist, who has been a godsend—and I mean that sincerely and literally. She was able to diagnose my son and knew what to do for treatment, including the meds that finally stabilized his mood.*

*I found out about educational advocacy training through my support group, too. Our school has been great for the most part, but my son's illness is so complicated that figuring out what he needs at school is a challenge. Now that I've been through the training, I can do a better job of helping with that, and if I have any questions, I know who to go to for answers.*

## FRIENDS AND FAMILY

You've probably already discovered that not everyone responds to your child with love, support, and understanding. People, even those closest to you, may blame you, openly criticize you and your child, and refuse to believe anything is truly wrong. Some may even try to sabotage your child's treatment. Relatives may be ashamed that it's a mental illness and mortified that you're "airing your dirty laundry in public."

These are not the friends and relatives you need as allies, no matter who they are or how close you used to be. Yes, you may be able to guide them to a better understanding of bipolar and what it means for your child—but right now, and on your team, you need people who already understand. People who've been there because their kids or grandkids have bipolar, too. People who empathize with the incredible effort it takes for you, day in and day out, to care for a chronically ill child. People who accept your child in all her complex, challenging glory.

Where do you find these people?

Some of them are already in your life: the grandparents who listen and run interference for you, the friend who isn't rattled by anything your child says or does. Others you'll meet through support groups, one of the most valuable resources available.

You might feel hesitant about joining a support group, worried that you'll have to reveal family secrets. It's hard enough to deal with your child's symptoms in the privacy of your own home without risking public shame. That's one of the reasons it's so easy for families dealing with bipolar to become isolated.

But navigating the bipolar maze as a solo traveler is extremely difficult, if not impossible. Getting to know other parents whose children have bipolar can make all the difference in the world.

Support groups are filled with parents who remember what it was like to feel alone, overwhelmed, and helpless as they watched their child suffer. They gather together—in person or online—to help each other with support, encouragement, advice, and lots of compassion. Many parents walk into their first support group meeting feeling ashamed and secretive about their child's illness, convinced that others will be horrified if they hear what their life is really like. What they discover is that every parent there tells the same story. They talk about the problems (and they are as bad as or worse than yours). They discuss ideas, strategies, and treatments that helped, and those that didn't. They share the names of their allies, the doctors, therapists, advocates, and others who have helped their families. They know your story because they're living it, too. You don't have to travel the maze alone.

*Michael's team includes grandparents from one side of his family but not the other.*

*After Michael was diagnosed, his parents discovered there were many relatives on one side of their family who had (or probably had) bipolar disorder. That side of the family guards its privacy; no one talks about mental illness. Anything that might indicate mental illness— the cousin with explosive rage, the uncle who drank too much, the rumored suicide—is ignored, denied, or blamed on something else: The cousin was a bad kid, the uncle a bum, the suicide only a rumor, never a fact.*

*The dynamics on the other side of the family are completely different. This side of the family is open and compassionate. Michael's grandma says they've all felt the "just give him a swat" impulse, but they know that Michael's a good kid, one who's gone through some awful things. They defend him to outsiders by calmly explaining that Michael has an illness, and that researchers are continuing to develop new and better treatments. They stay in touch with Michael and his parents through frequent phones calls, lots of e-mails, and visits several times a year. They provide a safe space when the clan gathers for holidays or a week or two in the summer. They talk about Michael's talents and gifts, and they provide much-needed respite for Michael's parents.*

*Michael's parents love and honor both sides of the family, and they also recognize that not everyone is able or willing to offer the acceptance and support they and Michael need.*

## FINDING THE RIGHT ALLIES

### WHERE TO BEGIN

The first step in getting help for your child is to speak with your child's primary care provider. Remember to take any records you've kept about your child's symptoms when you talk to the doctor. The doctor can rule out possible medical causes of the symptoms and refer you to a knowledgeable specialist in your area. If your child's symptoms are life-threatening—any behavior that endangers himself or others, including talking about or attempting suicide—your first step may be through the hospital emergency room.

You can find more recommendations for specialists from other parents, support groups, community healthcare directories, and reputable Web sites, such as www.bpkids.org and www.stepup4kids.com, that are dedicated to pediatric bipolar disorder. (Appendix E has a list of useful Web sites and other resources.) You should also check with your health insurance carrier for recommendations and to see which specialists are covered under your policy.

---

*Keri's team includes a family doctor; her "regular" psychiatrist; the psychiatrist, psychologist, teachers, and staff of the therapeutic residential school she attends; and her parents. Last year, it included doctors and staff at the emergency room, a psychiatric hospital, and her basketball coach.*

---

### SELECTING A SPECIALIST

What makes a psychiatrist a specialist?

Not all psychiatrists treat all types of mental illness. The same is true for advanced practice psychiatric nurses and every other potential ally.

Some specialize in adults, others in teens or young children.

Some specialize in particular illnesses—one psychiatrist might focus on bipolar, ADHD, and anxiety disorders; another on autism; yet another on schizophrenia or drug abuse.

Some psychiatrists and advanced practice nurses become experts in psychopharmacology. Their focus is on the medications used to treat mental illness. They have experience and in-depth knowledge about what meds are available, what the effects, side effects, and interactions with other meds are likely to be, and the best approaches for using medications. Other psychiatrists and advanced practice nurses focus primarily on therapy, support, and advocacy.

This doesn't mean each specialist doesn't know about the other illnesses, age groups, and treatments. It does mean that they've dedicated their careers to a particular illness or group of illnesses, age range, or treatment. Their continuing education, training, and clinical practice are focused, sometimes exclusively, on that particular subspecialty.

On your treatment team, you don't want just any specialist. You want a specialist who has experience with kids like yours: an expert who is up-to-date on bipolar and bipolar plus in kids in the same age range as yours. The psychiatric specialist you find might be one who focuses on therapy and support and who consults regularly with a colleague who's an expert on medications. Your psychiatric specialist might be the meds expert, with therapy, support, and advocacy coming through your therapeutic and educational allies. What ally comes from which category isn't as important as finding the right allies for your child.

To become an expert in one or more of these specialty areas doesn't happen overnight. After completing their education and training requirements, psychiatric (and other) specialists develop their expertise through two important avenues.

They gain extensive clinical experience over many years working with a particular category of patients (preschoolers with mood disorders or teens with substance abuse, for example).

Experts also keep up with cutting-edge research and changes in clinical practice that are rapidly and continuously advancing our knowledge and treatment options. This includes attending conferences where researchers share the latest results—the "breaking news" of psychiatry.

Even in this age of electronic communications, it can take months for research results to appear in reliable online journals. It can be two years or more before the information appears in the printed pages of a professional magazine. A specialist who waits for the printed report is an out-of-date specialist.

That's one of the reasons your family doctor may not know the latest about bipolar disorder. His specialty is family medicine, and his attention is focused on staying current with the research and practice of family medicine, not child and teen psychiatry.

You want treatment team members who are the most knowledgeable and up-to-date on the care that will benefit *your* child. That includes a family doctor who's current on family medicine. It's great if your family doctor is also familiar with mental illness in children and has a good working relationship with an appropriate psychiatric specialist—one whose expertise includes treating kids like yours and active involvement in conferences that present the latest findings about kids like yours.

Not sure if the professional you're talking to is the specialist you need? Ask! We work hard to develop our areas of expertise and even harder to keep them. We'll tell you what age groups we work with, what illnesses we focus on or treat most often, and what we do to stay current. Professionals aren't offended by these questions; we expect them.

Because so much of what we know about bipolar disorder in kids is new, few clinicians have the expert skills necessary to diagnose and treat bipolar. There's also a shortage of child psychiatrists, psychopharmacologists, and other psychiatric specialists. If you can't find an expert close to home, consider working with someone locally who meets most of your criteria and who will consult with a more experienced colleague. For example, in our clinics in Massachusetts, we evaluate kids, diagnose or confirm a diagnosis, and work with the child's "home" doctor to guide treatment for kids who live as far away as Japan.

After you have a good recommendation or two, it's time to talk. Sometimes, parents feel uncomfortable asking specialists about their qualifications, but it really isn't much different from asking anyone whose services you need. You wouldn't hire someone to replace your roof without checking his references and experience; you need to do the same for the specialists you hire for your child's care.

Ultimately, you want to establish a relationship with a clinician you trust. That relationship begins now, by asking questions and listening to the answers. Ask:

- What area of psychiatry do you specialize in?

- Have you worked with children in the same age range as my child?

- Do you regularly attend conferences and lectures to stay up-to-date on research and changes in clinical practice related to bipolar and bipolar plus? What else do you do to stay current?

- Are you accepting new patients or are you available only to evaluate or consult on my child's case? How soon are you available?

- What costs are involved? Does my health insurance cover some or all of the cost? If not, what are the fee structures?

- What are your approaches to evaluation and treatment?

Listen carefully to the replies. Do the specialist's comments and questions convey a sense that she really understands what you're experiencing at home? Beware of professionals who begin to blame you, even if they seem sincere and well-meaning. Comments like, "It seems hard for you to handle Sara's behavior" miss the point. Of course it's hard—does this specialist have any idea what it's like to be pummeled by a raging, out-of-control eight-year-old?

Listen for active solutions that aren't glib. There is no "one way" or "single right answer" to treat anything in psychiatry, especially an illness as challenging as bipolar disorder. Your specialist should say something like, "Well, there are a number of different approaches we can take. Let's think about them together and go over the pros and cons."

## A MATTER OF STYLE

A specialist can be perfectly qualified and still not be the best choice for your team simply because of her personal style. We like to use ourselves to demonstrate this.

Janet is high-energy, intense, and direct. Her speech is rapid-fire and she tends to lean forward when she talks, as if she's urging you on. She asks and answers questions quickly.

Mary Ann is mellower. She tends to sit back in her chair as if she has all the time in the world. Her voice is softer, she speaks more slowly than Janet, and she pauses a bit before saying anything.

We both have a lot of experience in treating kids who have bipolar disorder. We cover about the same amount of ground in an appointment. We both work with younger kids and teens, though Mary Ann tends to do more psychotherapy as well as meds management and Janet works with more research subjects.

For some, Janet's a good match; for others, Mary Ann's a

better choice. This isn't a matter of what's right or wrong; it's a matter of style.

Remember, you need a specialist you can trust and understand. If, despite all the evidence claiming this expert is practically perfect, you can't establish that comfort level, find a different specialist. The best expert in the world won't help if you can't communicate.

> *Matt's team includes a pediatrician, an advanced practice psychiatric nurse, a therapist, an educational advocate, his uncle, and his mom.*

## THE FIRST APPOINTMENT: WHAT TO EXPECT

When we accept a new patient, we usually talk with parents first, without the child present. When you bring your child in for the first time, we perform a diagnostic evaluation, assess your child's level of safety and functioning, and talk about what we think is going on and what the next steps will be. These initial appointments typically take about sixty to ninety minutes, sometimes longer.

Why separate appointments?

Many kids with bipolar disorder can't recognize that their moods and behaviors are symptoms of a disorder. Their lack of insight is, in fact, a common part of the symptom mix.

They rationalize and blame others to explain their behavior ("He started it!" or "I'd be fine if she'd get off my back!"). Extreme irritability, low tolerance for frustration, difficulty expressing feelings, shaky problem-solving skills, and impulsivity combine to form a volatile mix. No matter how carefully you phrase your report about your child's moods and behavior, there's an excellent chance that he's going to interpret anything you say as an insult, criticism, or unfair attack.

Of course, it isn't just the bipolar symptoms that make it difficult for your child to listen to a discussion of his symptoms. Most kids with bipolar already feel victimized, demoralized, and misunderstood, which makes them even more sensitive to perceived criticism. It's common for them to react defensively to your reports, from protesting their innocence to storming out of the office.

This kind of aggravation doesn't help anyone. So we begin by meeting with you, the parent or parents. We meet with your son or daughter later, either immediately following our first meeting with you or at another time.

When we observe and talk with kids during an appointment, we'll usually catch hints of what's going on, but most kids don't exhibit strong symptoms during office visits. From the very beginning, we rely on your observations to get an accurate picture.

Your observations include the records you've kept concerning your child's moods, thinking, and emotions (the same records we talked about in Chapter 5). Be prepared to answer detailed questions about your child's history, too. Bring notes or records about your child's

> *development* (did he meet, beat, or miss developmental milestones?);
> *medical history* (has your child been diagnosed with any illnesses or medical problems [bipolar, plus disorders, other medical illnesses of any kind])? have you tried meds? what ones? what doses? what was the effect? any side effects?);
> *family history* (any brain disorders, including bipolar, depression, or alcoholism, in other family members? any other illnesses, such as heart disease or diabetes? any history of how other family members have responded to medications?);

*results of any previous testing;*
*social interactions and any academic or learning issues;* and
*other significant events or concerns.*

Be as specific and open as you can about your observations.
Your doctor won't be shocked that your ten-year-old has
knocked holes in the walls or that your four-year-old has been
expelled from every preschool in the county. It's all part of the
picture that helps us figure out what is going on with your
child and what to do about it to help.

At the first meeting between your child and the doctor
and for most appointments after, you'll be there, too, especially if your child is young. As your child grows, you may
gradually reach a time when it makes more sense for the doctor to meet with you and your child separately. As long as your
child is a minor under your care, you have access to any information from your child's appointments.

Sometimes, we can make a diagnosis during the first visit.
Other times, the picture is more complicated and we'll need to
gather more information before we can make an accurate
diagnosis. We'll also decide what the best treatment setting
will be. Outpatient is our first choice, but if your child is in
danger of hurting himself or others, he may need to be
treated in an inpatient hospital until he's better stabilized.

After diagnosis, you and your child's clinician will discuss
treatment options. Between now and the next appointment,
you'll continue to track your child's symptoms. At subsequent
appointments (which usually take less time than the initial
evaluation), your observations will help identify whether the
treatment you're trying is making a difference.

### HOW TO BUILD A TEAM IN SIX EASY STEPS

1. Talk to your family doctor first; rule out medical causes.
2. Get referrals—from your family doctor, support groups, reputable online sources, insurance company.
3. Ask questions! (Experience with kids like yours? Up-to-date?)
4. Listen to the answers and other comments. (Communication style? Acknowledges your concerns? Supports your efforts to find solutions for your child? Suggests exploring various treatment options?)
5. Add or subtract team members as needed. If a team member turns out to be a bad match, replace him.
6. Keep good records and open lines of communication so that information can get from one team member to another when necessary and appropriate.

*Chapter 7*

# TREATMENT TWISTS AND TURNS

## FINDING THE BEST TREATMENT FOR YOUR CHILD

*There are lots of good moments in life, lots of bad moments. You could have one day with lots of good, or a bad day with thirty-six temper tantrums in an hour. I've gotten used to taking meds. I don't mind it much. I know I'll always have to take them.*

*My advice to other kids is to stay confident. Don't worry about the fact that you have a brain disorder. Don't be ashamed; it's okay. Everyone is unique. You'll still be smart. You'll be taking medicine. Don't be afraid—I'm not. Stay confident.*

MICHAEL, AGE TEN, DIAGNOSED AGE SEVEN

Now that you know what you're dealing with, what do you do?

Pediatric bipolar disorder is a complex illness, so it's not surprising that treatment can be complex, too. We regard every child diagnosed in our clinics as a unique person with a unique version of bipolar disorder. Treating the child's condition is therefore a unique challenge.

As the leader of your child's treatment team, you have many decisions to make.

The first is not *how* to treat the illness, but *whether* to treat it. No matter how much you love your child, no matter how determined you are to find the best help for her, you may still be leery about treating your child's illness with medication, with good cause. The drugs commonly used are powerful and useful, but they carry the risk of side effects, which in rare cases can be serious. The media are full of conflicting reports about mental illness and medication, and celebrities weigh in with divergent claims about treatment. Social and political forces present the symptoms of mental illness as signs of a "weak character" or a "bad kid in need of a good swat." Healthcare providers who have little experience with early-onset bipolar disorder accuse parents of dodging responsibility when they blame their child's behavior on the illness. Experts disagree and complicated research results are confusing and seem to contradict each other. It's no wonder parents hesitate to treat their kids.

Sometimes parents are reluctant to have their children use medications because they want to believe that the illness really isn't that bad: "If we try harder, or give him more vitamins, or wait for her to grow a little more..." the thinking goes.

But as we know from hard clinical experience, failing to treat bipolar disorder carries enormous risks.

There's the risk that your teen with bipolar may become involved in dangerous, possibly criminal, behavior during a manic episode and land in a complicated legal system that is often unsympathetic toward mental illness. There's the risk that your child may succumb to substance abuse (often an attempt at self-medication) and addiction. There's the risk that your child will develop additional disorders and the risk of health complications because he can't take care of himself or she places herself in unsafe situations. There's the terrible risk of suicide: As many as 18% of untreated children die by suicide before their eighteenth birthdays.

We know that children with untreated bipolar disorder often miss critical developmental milestones because the symptoms derail their progress through the normal stages of childhood. They risk academic failure because the illness interferes with their ability to think and learn. Their symptoms lead to many absences from school. They may be sequestered in programs that focus on behavioral challenges at the expense of academic progress. They aren't able to participate in spring soccer, Little League, and other extracurricular programs. These kids are at risk for social failure and isolation, too, because their peers single out or ostracize the child whose behavior is odd.

There are two hard truths about bipolar disorder. First, like any chronic illness, it will almost certainly get worse if it is left untreated. Second, treatment, while usually effective, is not perfect. It takes time to find the best treatment for each individual, there may be side effects, and there is no known cure for the disorder at this time.

There are also two big hopes about bipolar disorder. First, with skill and perseverance, you and your team can develop a successful treatment strategy for your child. Second, research into the causes and treatments of pediatric bipolar disorder is rapidly expanding our understanding of this illness, leading to improved treatment now and someday, we hope, a cure.

If your daughter has been diagnosed with bipolar disorder (with or without other disorders) and you're still debating whether or not to seek treatment, consider this:

If your child had a chronic *physical* illness—diabetes or cerebral palsy or cancer, for example—would you withhold or delay treatment for her? Most likely, you and she would work together every day to find and use the best possible balance of medicine, therapy, support, and appropriate complementary treatments to help her grow and thrive despite that illness.

Treating a child who has a chronic *mental* illness requires exactly the same approach.

\* \* \*

In this chapter, we'll guide you through the twists and turns of treatment options. As you make your way through this part of the maze, you'll learn about the types of medications used to treat bipolar in children and teens. You'll discover why your doctor might recommend one drug over another to try first and why your child might need more than one medication.

Along the way, you'll meet kids like yours who show you how the treatment process worked with them and their families. As you finish this chapter, you may be surprised to realize that you've learned to think like a doctor or nurse practitioner—you'll understand the how and why of your child's treatment.

Of course, treatment is more than just medicine. You, your family, and your child may need therapy and other support over time. There are different kinds of therapy and support, just as there are different kinds of medicine. You'll find descriptions of the ones most often used in treating bipolar in Chapter 8.

---

### WARNING!
Do not start or stop any medication without first checking with your clinician!

Changing any treatment—starting or stopping a medication, adjusting dosage, and making other alterations—must be done carefully and under the guidance of a medical professional in order to minimize risks and get the best results for your child.

---

## WHAT TO EXPECT: MEDS AND KIDS

We usually begin treatment for pediatric bipolar disorder with one or more drugs that help bring the most life-disrupting symptoms under control. Once your child's bipolar disorder is stabilized, we may decide to add other medications to treat plus problems, ADHD, for example. Nonmedication therapies will probably be part of your child's treatment plan, too.

It's important to remember that every child is unique, and every child's response to medication is unique. There's no way to identify how a child will respond to a particular medication other than by trying the medication. What works wonders for one child may make no difference or make things worse for another. Sometimes, this can make you feel like you're using your kid as a guinea pig. Oh this didn't work, let's try that, or that, or *that*. It seems random at best and terrifying at worst.

But treatment really isn't random. There's a logical approach based on research and clinical experience, combined with what you know about your child, his symptoms, your family history, and other information. We work hard to find the right combination of drugs, therapy, and support for your child that will give you all relief.

Trying a medication is always a balance between "start low and go slow" and "hurry, make it work *now.*" Starting with a low dosage and gradually increasing the amount of medication helps minimize side effects or avoid them altogether. It also lets us find the lowest effective dose and helps prevent giving too much medicine. The goal is to give your child enough medication to help, but not so much that she is overmedicated or suffering from side effects.

When there is enough of a medicine in the body to make a noticeable difference in symptoms, the drug has reached *therapeutic levels*. For some drugs, this is determined by checking the results of a blood test. More often, the therapeutic level is found by trial—observing that a particular dose is the one that brings the most improvement for your child with the fewest side effects. Most drugs used to treat bipolar have a recommended starting dose and a range where they work best.

How long it takes to get from the starting dose to

therapeutic levels is different for different drugs, individual circumstances, unique patient reactions, and clinician preference. You might see an improvement in your child's symptoms within days, or not for many weeks. Even if there's a good response to a medication early on, it may take two to four weeks or longer to be sure that this particular drug or combination of drugs and this particular dose is what works best for your child. Your child might continue to do well on that medication, or his symptoms might reappear in a few weeks or months, and he'll need to try a different dose or a different medication.

For example, lithium is one of the drugs used to stabilize mood. If we decide to treat your son with lithium, we'll generally begin with a low dose, 150 or 300 milligrams per day, and gradually increase the dose. After at least five days on a prescribed dose, we measure the actual level of the drug in the blood twelve hours after the last dose. If the lithium hasn't reached therapeutic levels yet, we gradually increase the dose as needed and recheck the blood levels after another five days. Once the blood tests show that the lithium has reached therapeutic levels, the dose stays the same, assuming that it is alleviating his symptoms and he isn't having too much trouble with side effects. After that, we monitor the lithium level and thyroid and kidney functioning by doing blood tests at least twice a year.

The process of finding the optimal dose can take several weeks, and symptoms often won't begin to improve until the lithium levels enter the therapeutic range. In other words, for the first couple of weeks it looks like the medication isn't working, and then, sometimes gradually, sometimes all of a sudden, the lithium "kicks in" and symptoms improve.

Here's another example. The drug Risperdal is one of a new group of medications called *atypical antipsychotics*. We've learned through both research and experience with kids at our clinics that these medications work as mood stabilizers, too, often more quickly than lithium, and are especially effective in easing rage storms, aggression, and reckless behavior. If your son is struggling with symptoms like these, we might try Risperdal or another atypical antipsychotic instead of lithium. His starting dose of Risperdal would be anywhere from 0.25 milligram to 1.0 milligram, depending on his symptoms—what they are and how severe they are; his history, including how he's reacted to other medications; and other factors. Even at a low dose, you may notice that symptoms begin to ease up within days after beginning Risperdal. As the dose increases, his symptoms may improve even more. At still higher doses, there might be more improvement without problems from side effects; or side effects might outweigh any additional improvement; or the symptoms might stay the same, with or without side effects. As the dose is slowly increased, you'll track the results, and your child's clinician will adjust the dosage based on your son's results and tolerance of the medication. Even though your son's initial response happened early, it may still take several weeks before you find the dose that works the best for him. And of course, Risperdal may not work at all, in which case, your doctor will try a different medication, going through the same process.

"Start low and go slow" also applies to adding, changing, and dropping medications. We add or adjust one medication at a time so we can tell whether it is making a difference or causing a side effect. Then its dosage is gradually adjusted until symptoms improve.

There is an exception to the "start low and go slow" rule: If your child is extremely ill and has been hospitalized, the clinician may add more than one medication at a time and increase the doses more rapidly, all while closely monitoring your child.

When a medication isn't working, your child should *not* stop taking the medication all at once unless it's an emergency, for example, a severe adverse reaction. You'll need to taper the medication—"go slow to get low"—before finally discontinuing that drug.

Sometimes, it's necessary to *cross-taper* medications. This means that while we're slowly *increasing* the dose of one medication, we're slowly *decreasing* the dose of another one. The two medications are usually the same *category* of drug, both atypical antipsychotics, for example, but one is either ineffective or causing side effects. Cross-tapering lets us slowly eliminate the drug that isn't working, which minimizes the chances of withdrawal symptoms. At the same time, we're working up to the therapeutic levels of the new medication and can tell more quickly if it is helping than if we waited until the first medication was completely discontinued.

It can take several weeks for a medication to completely clear out from your child's system. Stopping a medication abruptly can result in serious withdrawal symptoms, may cause other symptoms to worsen, and may increase the risk of suicide.

So remember: Whether starting or stopping, go slowly.


## PHARMACOGENETICS

Today, research results, clinical experience, and the information you provide help your treatment team identify what treatment is most likely to be effective for your child, but there's no way to be sure what will work until treatment begins. Current research is exploring how to make this process faster and more accurate by matching treatments to an individual's genome. Someday, a needle prick and genetic analysis may tell us exactly which medications to use.

## THE BASIC MEDS MAP

There's a set of steps that clinicians follow when they recommend medication or other treatment for bipolar disorder. The twists and turns happen in treatment because your child may have to try several different medications before finding the ones that work best.

Figure 4 shows the basic path you and your child will travel to find the right medications. As you can see, the path returns to "Does it help?" every time, until you find a treatment that does help, with as few side effects as possible.

Notice that as you travel the twists and turns, it's quite possible that your child will end up taking more than one medication. In fact, most children and teens with bipolar need to take several medications. This can be alarming to someone who doesn't have experience in treating bipolar, including other doctors and school personnel.

The rest of this section tells you about the specific medications most often used to treat bipolar in children and teens. You can begin by reading through these descriptions, or you can skip over this part and head straight into the stories of families and their experiences, which begin on page 172, returning here when you want to know more about a particular medication. For more details on a specific drug, including potential side effects, check the tables in Appendix D.

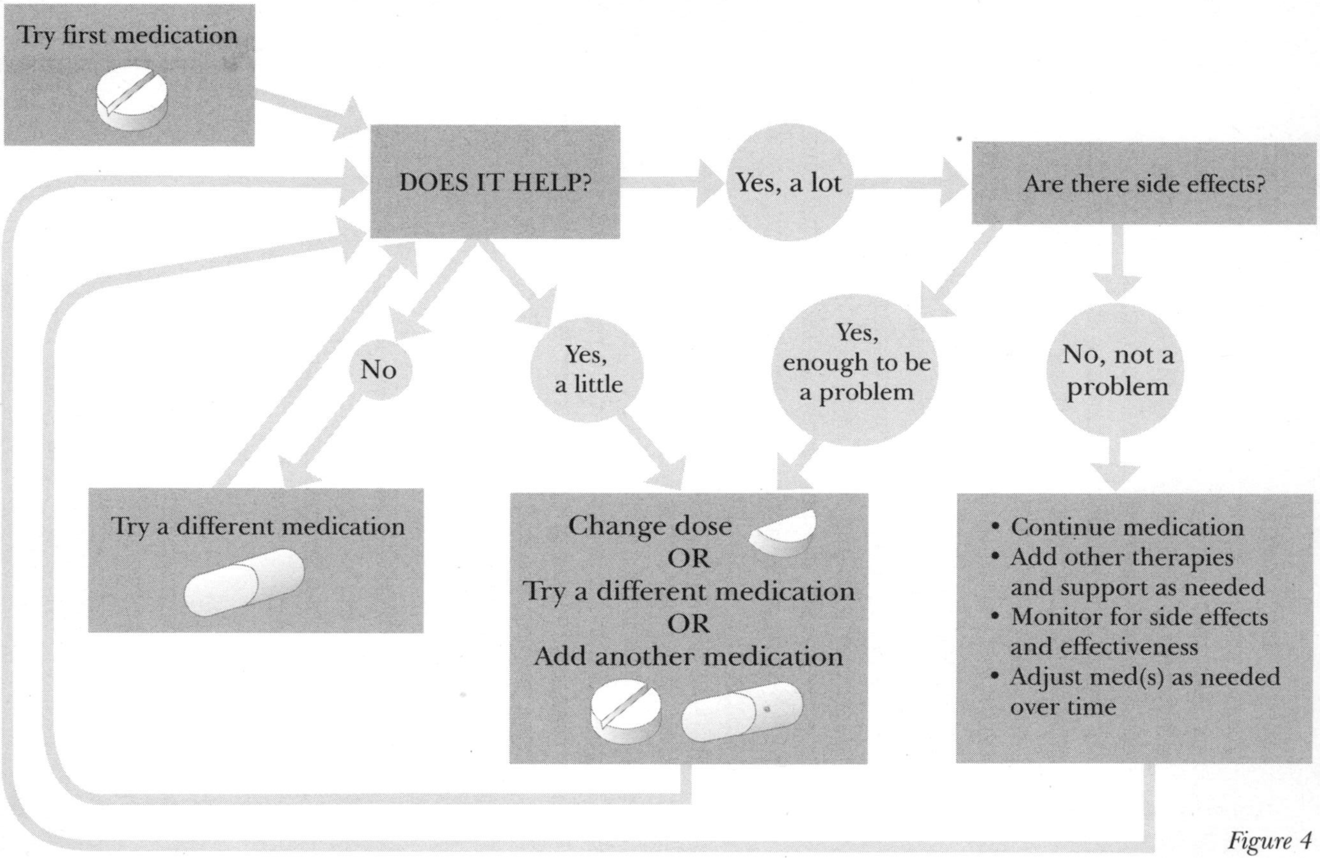

Try first medication

DOES IT HELP?

Yes, a lot

Are there side effects?

No, not a problem

Yes, enough to be a problem

Yes, a little

No

Change dose
OR
Try a different medication
OR
Add another medication

Try a different medication

- Continue medication
- Add other therapies and support as needed
- Monitor for side effects and effectiveness
- Adjust med(s) as needed over time

*Figure 4*

## "OFF-LABEL" AND THE FDA

What is commonly referred to as "FDA approval" is really shorthand for "proven safe and effective" enough that the drug can be marketed for the specified application. The FDA doesn't approve drugs or tests for all uses, and it doesn't recommend treatments. That's your doctor's responsibility. The FDA examines the studies that show whether a particular drug is *safe* (including the potential for minor, major, or dangerous side effects) and *effective* (the drug does what it claims to do).

Many drugs developed to treat specific conditions are later discovered to be useful in treating entirely different conditions. Anticonvulsants are one example. They were originally developed to treat seizure disorders and, like any new drug, went through clinical trials testing their safety and effectiveness. These studies provided the evidence the FDA required to issue its approval for their use in treating seizures.

When a drug has FDA approval for one condition and a clinician prescribes it to treat another condition, this is called an *off-label* use.

Parents sometimes worry that using a drug that doesn't have FDA approval for treating their child's bipolar disorder means that the drug might not be safe. Sometimes they question whether the medication can be effective since it wasn't invented to treat this particular problem.

The safety of the drug is the same, regardless of which illness it is being used for. It also has the same potential for side effects. If the FDA has approved a medication as safe and effective for one use, that drug is generally equally safe for an off-label use.

Many of the medications used to treat bipolar disorder were first used to treat the adult-onset form of the illness, and most of the research on safety and effectiveness has been done with adults. Since children and teens may respond differently to a drug than adults do, it's important to continue research that evaluates safety and effectiveness in kids. Pharmaceutical companies have incentives to do this; for example, they may be able to extend the life of their patent for a medication.

The FDA establishes safety by reviewing extensive research studies that examine the drug in a specific population and age group. Researchers analyze information from these studies to understand how the drug works, what side effects are associated with it, and how safe it is in the age group or gender studied. It takes additional research and clinical experience to know if the drug will be similarly safe and effective in another group.

Discovering that a drug may be effective for off-label uses begins in many ways, sometimes serendipitously. Ultimately, research studies combined with clinical results confirm or refute that usefulness. Whether or not those results make their way through the expensive and time-consuming FDA review process is more a question of finances than one of safety and effectiveness.

Many research studies that explore a new use for an existing drug are small or continue for only a short time, so they don't provide the volume of data that the FDA requires, and the wealth of information gathered through clinical practice that supports the safety and effectiveness of an off-label use isn't from a formal research study. This is especially true for many drugs that are now considered standard treatments for childhood psychiatric disorders.

Sometimes drugs produce unexpected effects—for example, antidepressants may trigger mania or stimulants may make bipolar symptoms worse—but this is not because the safety and side effects are different for off-label use. Antidepressants are "approved" for treating depression and stimulants are "approved" for treating ADHD. If these conditions exist along with mania, then neither the antidepressant nor the stimulant will work as expected.

This is why an accurate, comprehensive diagnosis is so important.

As we go to press, the only medications with FDA approval for pediatric bipolar disorder are lithium, which is approved for use down to age twelve, and Risperdal (risperidone), approved for use down to age ten. Many more are undergoing the approval process.

## MOOD-STABILIZING DRUGS

If we'd been practicing medicine a hundred years ago, we wouldn't have had an effective treatment for bipolar disorder. Fifty years ago, there was just one, lithium, and if it didn't help, there weren't any alternatives. Now there are lots of choices, with more being developed and tested every year.

The first kind of medication we use in treating bipolar disorder is a *mood stabilizer*. As the name implies, mood stabilizers help control the extreme mood changes of bipolar.

There are three categories for mood stabilizers: lithium, anticonvulsants, and atypical antipsychotics.

Lithium, the first mood stabilizer commonly used to treat bipolar disorder in adults, is still used in both children and adults. Its first recorded use was in ancient Greece, by the physician Galen. In modern times, Australian psychiatrist John Cade described in 1948 that lithium helped calm manic patients. In 1974, the FDA approved lithium to treat acute mania and for the long-term prevention of manic episodes.

Beginning in the 1970s, neurologists and researchers discovered that certain drugs used to treat seizure disorders improved mood stability. These medications, called *anticonvulsants,* often helped the symptoms of patients who didn't respond to lithium. They also helped those who had rapid cycling or mixed mood states—the "spinning star" that kids often have.

In the 1990s, research showed that bipolar disorder in children and adults also responded well to a new class of antipsychotic medications. These *atypical antipsychotics* (also called *novel* or *second-generation* antipsychotics) are now classified as mood stabilizers. All of the medications in this class have received FDA approval for treating bipolar disorder in adults, and they all have scientific evidence supporting their usefulness in treating bipolar in children.

Depending on symptoms, response to each medication, and the presence of other illnesses and disorders, we may prescribe a single mood stabilizer, one mood stabilizer used in combination with one or more other mood stabilizers, or mood stabilizers used together with other kinds of medication.

## LITHIUM

Lithium is the granddaddy of mood stabilizers. It was initially used to treat acute mania in adults. Over time, doctors and patients realized that it also helped to prevent the cycles of bipolar disorder. Lithium is FDA-approved for treating bipolar disorder in those who are twelve years old and older.

Lithium works well for 70%–80% of adults who have bipolar disorder, and it's effective for about 50% of children and teens. Whether lithium works may be partly genetic; if a parent with bipolar responds well to lithium treatment, there's a greater chance that the child with bipolar will also respond well. Lithium may not be the best choice for treating rapid-cycling bipolar—the spinning star. For these patients, we usually begin with one of the other mood stabilizers. Depending on how the child responds, we might add lithium later as part of the treatment, or switch to lithium.

Side effects range from the minor and manageable, for example increased thirst, to the serious, such as kidney problems and lithium toxicity. Children who don't tolerate lithium well will need to try a different mood stabilizer.

In addition, treating with lithium means frequent blood tests. These tests monitor kidney and thyroid function and make sure the lithium level is in the therapeutic range and not rising to toxic levels. This can limit lithium's usefulness, especially for kids who have an extra hard time with needles and blood draws.

Your child's lithium levels can fluctuate in response to fluids, salt (sodium), and anything that affects kidney function. If your daughter is an avid soccer player and gets dehydrated during an intense game, the lithium level in her blood will increase and it may reach toxic levels. If she drinks too much water, her blood may become diluted and the lithium levels may drop below the therapeutic range.

If your son comes down with a nasty bug that causes fluid loss—fever, vomiting, or diarrhea—his lithium levels may rise as he becomes dehydrated (his blood has less fluid so the lithium is more concentrated) and become toxic. The nasty bug doesn't have to be one that causes an upset tummy. William, one of the six-year-olds we see every month, had an ear infection. His mother called 911 when William began stumbling around as if he were drunk and wasn't able to speak clearly. At the emergency room, they tested his lithium levels, which were too high. The ER staff suspected that the lithium levels had gone up because the antibiotic William was taking for his ear infection may have slowed down the rate his kidneys were excreting the lithium. Ibuprofen (Advil, Motrin, Nuprin) can have this effect, too.

Some doctors prefer to try lithium first in treating early-onset bipolar disorder because it's been used successfully in many people for a long time, or they might choose it if there is a family history of good lithium response. Others prefer to begin with another type of mood stabilizer (an anticonvulsant or atypical antipsychotic). If your child's symptoms are severe and include psychosis, your doctor may begin treatment with a combination of mood stabilizers, perhaps lithium or an anticonvulsant plus one of the atypical antipsychotics.

ANTICONVULSANTS

Next on the mood-stabilizer scene, used since the 1970s, are several anticonvulsants. We use two of these, valproate (Depakote) and carbamazepine (Tegretol, Carbatrol, Equetro), instead of or in addition to lithium and atypical antipsychotics. Both require careful monitoring of blood levels. Depakote can affect the liver and pancreas and may lead to the development of polycystic ovaries. Carbamazepine can affect the bone marrow's production of white blood cells.

We might use oxcarbazepine (Trileptal), another anticonvulsant, if these first-line choices don't work, but we usually don't begin with Trileptal because research on its use in kids is not so encouraging. It may be effective in some adults and children and is easier to use because it has fewer side effects than its cousin, carbamazepine. Unfortunately, it appears to be less effective than carbamazepine.

Lamotrigine (Lamictal) is another anticonvulsant that we use in treating pediatric bipolar disorder, especially in adolescents. It's FDA-approved for treating bipolar depression in adults and is gaining clinical acceptance in treating bipolar depression in teens, too. Studies examining its use in younger children are under way.

Some anticonvulsants that are not effective in treating bipolar disorder may be useful in treating some of the plus problems of bipolar plus and for treating side effects from other medications. These include gabapentin (Neurontin), which may be used to treat anxiety, and the benzodiazepines, such as clonazepam (Klonopin) and lorazepam (Ativan), used for both anxiety and seizures.

Anticonvulsants have some potentially serious side effects, including liver problems, blood disorders, and cognitive (thinking) difficulties. More common and less serious side effects include dry mouth, drowsiness, and changes in appetite or weight (up or down).

## ATYPICAL ANTIPSYCHOTICS

Atypical antipsychotics, which include the brands Abilify, Clozaril, Geodon, Invega, Risperdal, Seroquel, and Zyprexa, are now our first choice in many cases for treating the acute mania and mood swings of bipolar disorder in children and teens because they work quickly and have a much lower risk of side effects compared to conventional or first-generation antipsychotics. Parents tell us that symptoms begin to improve within a few days to a few weeks, compared to the many weeks often required for other meds. The atypical antipsychotics have also turned out to be especially useful in easing rage storms, aggression, agitation, and reckless behavior, which are all common in pediatric bipolar.

These drugs, also called *atypical neuroleptics, second-generation antipsychotics,* or *novel antipsychotics,* were developed to overcome the severe side effects that older antipsychotic medications (drugs such as Haldol, Thorazine, Mellaril, and Trilafon) caused.

Although atypical antipsychotics work quickly and have fewer side effects than the older antipsychotics, they are not risk-free. One of the more distressing side effects associated with these medications is a significant increase in appetite and weight gain. The weight gain is probably caused by a combination of slower basal metabolic rate (which means the body uses fewer calories) and the drug's effect on the hypothalamus (the part of the brain that tells you to eat when you're hungry and to stop eating when you're full). Some atypical antipsychotics may change the body's sensitivity to leptin, a hormone that helps regulate body weight, metabolism, and reproductive function. Other factors may increase susceptibility to type 2 diabetes.

In addition to blood tests monitoring glucose, cholesterol, and triglycerides (and with some medications, prolactin levels), your clinician will follow your child's height and weight and monitor him for involuntary movements. Tardive dyskinesia, a neurological condition characterized by potentially permanent writhing movements around the nose, mouth, and tongue, was a common and often disfiguring side effect of the older antipsychotic medications. It appears to be rare with atypical antipsychotics, but you and your clinician still need to watch for these kinds of movements. Other muscle spasms can also occur with these medications, which can be alarming but are not permanent or dangerous. Be sure to tell your clinician right away if you notice anything.

Often, we will select a particular atypical antipsychotic *because* of the kind of side effects it's likely to have. For example, if your son is overweight or you have a strong family history of diabetes, we will begin treatment with an atypical antipsychotic that is less likely to make him gain weight. If he's underweight, we might not worry about prescribing a medication that has a higher chance of causing weight gain.

Not everyone who takes the same atypical antipsychotic gains weight or develops an increased risk for diabetes (with or without weight gain), nor do all atypical antipsychotics have the same set of side effects. As with all drugs used to treat bipolar disorder, your son's response will determine whether a particular drug is appropriate for him.

One of the atypical antipsychotics, clozapine (Clozaril) is a medication of last resort for pediatric bipolar disorder because it carries a risk of life-threatening blood dyscrasia (a blood disease that can cause neutropenia, a life-threatening decrease in white blood cells). However, this medication can be remarkably effective for some children, and regular monitoring can keep the potential blood dyscrasia from becoming life-threatening. We use it when none of the other treatments has helped, monitoring its safety through blood tests every week or two.

## OTHER MEDICATIONS

The medications described next are *not* first-line treatments for bipolar disorder in kids. We use these drugs to manage specific symptoms (especially short-term, during a crisis) and to treat side effects and some of the plus problems of bipolar plus. In general, we prescribe them in addition to one or more of the mood stabilizers described above. They include antidepressants, benzodiazepines, and conventional antipsychotics.

### ANTIDEPRESSANTS

At first, it seems logical that antidepressants should be useful in treating bipolar disorder; after all, depression is part of the illness.

But the same antidepressants that can alleviate major depressive disorder (or *unipolar depression disorder*)—what many people call clinical or severe depression—can trigger mania, hypomania, or an increased rate of cycling in someone who has bipolar disorder. As many as half of the children who have not had symptoms of mania but show signs of or develop severe depression before puberty ultimately develop bipolar disorder, so our concern about triggering mania is important.

Yet antidepressants *are* often an important part of treatment for bipolar disorder *after the mania is stabilized.* We introduce antidepressants slowly and carefully in order to treat any residual depression without triggering mania. For example, when Becky was thirteen, her parents brought her to us for an evaluation because she was irritable all the time. She said mean things to the kids at school, and the other girls retaliated and excluded her. She screamed at her mother at the slightest provocation. Becky was also sad and lonely and no longer interested in extracurricular activities. Risperdal brought her mania (the extreme irritability and rage) under control, but it wasn't until we added an antidepressant that Becky began to join in the after-school activities that she'd always loved.

These medications include the selective serotonin reuptake inhibitors (SSRIs), such as fluoxetine (Prozac), paroxetine (Paxil), citalopram (Celexa), fluvoxamine (Luvox), and sertraline (Zoloft); the selective norepinephrine reuptake inhibitors (SNRIs), such as venlafaxine (Effexor); and the atypical antidepressant bupropion (Wellbutrin).

For some children, adjusting the dosage and types of anticonvulsants or atypical antipsychotics may resolve the depression without the use of antidepressants. Robin, another thirteen-year-old girl, had symptoms similar to Becky's. In Robin's case, a combination of three mood stabilizers (Trileptal, Risperdal, and lithium) remedied the bipolar symptoms and, after we tweaked dosages, the depression, too.

We are using the anticonvulsant lamotrigine (Lamictal) more and more often to treat bipolar depression in kids, especially teens. The worry with Lamictal is the risk of a serious rash called Stevens-Johnson syndrome, so we usually try a different medication first. When we do use Lamictal, we start with a low dose and increase it very gradually, which decreases the chances of developing the Stevens-Johnson rash side effect.

Some clinicians think that if you have bipolar disorder, you should never take an antidepressant because of the risk that it will make the mania worse. You'll need to discuss the pros and cons with your clinician to determine what's best for your child.

There are several nondrug approaches for treating depression that may be appropriate for some children and teens.

These are described in "Other Medical Therapies" later in this section and in Chapter 8. (See pages 165 and 196.)

## BENZODIAZEPINES

Benzodiazepines are minor tranquilizers. They're used to treat anxiety disorders and some seizures.

In adults who have bipolar disorder, benzodiazepines are used to treat acute mania and the side effects of antipsychotic medications. They can also reduce anxiety, agitation, and sleep problems. But there is not much research on using benzodiazepines in children and teens. In some younger children, these drugs may increase, not reduce, mania, agitation, and anxiety. In addition, benzodiazepines carry a risk of dependency, and they may result in too much sedation and problems with thinking and learning.

Because of these concerns, we typically give benzodiazepines to children and teens only for a short time, often at the beginning of treatment with mood stabilizers. Once the mood stabilizers are working, we discontinue the benzodiazepines. If the child still has a lot of anxiety, we might continue prescribing a benzodiazepine until we can establish a different antianxiety medication. And, for some kids, long-term use of benzodiazepines is just the right treatment.

## CONVENTIONAL ANTIPSYCHOTICS

Conventional or first-generation antipsychotics were developed to treat schizophrenia. These medications are called *major tranquilizers* and can be extremely sedating. Their use has expanded to include treatment for several other illnesses, including bipolar disorder. Because of their side effects, we use most conventional antipsychotics only for short-term treatment or if symptoms don't respond to other treatments. Although the conventional antipsychotics are less expensive than the newer atypical antipsychotics, we actually know less about how effective they are for pediatric bipolar disorder. A major concern with them is that their side-effect profiles are worse, especially if they are used for a long time.

In the short run, people treated with conventional antipsychotics may appear to have an illness that looks like Parkinson's disorder, with stiffness, a shuffling gait, and a masked or frozen facial expression. In the long run, people treated with these older medications may develop tardive dyskinesia, a potentially permanent and disfiguring disorder with involuntary movements that commonly occur around the mouth, lips, and tongue. These movement problems may also occur with the atypical antipsychotics, but far less often and with less severity.

## BIPOLAR AND BIPOLAR PLUS: HIERARCHY OF TREATMENT

Sometimes, treating bipolar disorder seems like squeezing a balloon: Squeeze in one place and a bulge shows up in another place. Medication alleviates your daughter's rage and temper tantrums, but her anxiety flares up. Or medication dampens her mood swings, but the teacher sends home notes complaining that she can't sit still and isn't paying attention.

Each child is unique: Each has a unique set of symptoms and unique reactions to treatment. When all symptoms are effectively treated, the balloon won't bulge.

It's important to remember that when you're dealing with bipolar plus, the bipolar disorder must be treated first. Treating your son's plus problems without treating his bipolar disorder can cause even more severe bipolar symptoms in him (for example, when antidepressants or stimulants trigger mania) and can shift or worsen the symptoms of the plus problems he suffers from.

Most children and teens with bipolar disorder have multiple problems and complex symptoms. Treatment tackles these one at a time, in a specific sequence or hierarchy. The hierarchy for the most common problems associated with bipolar disorder is:

| | |
|---|---|
| **Treat First:** | Mania |
| **Treat Second:** | Depression |
| **Treat Third:** | Anxiety or ADHD, depending on which is causing the most difficulty for the child |

## MEDICATIONS FOR PLUS PROBLEMS

Once a child's bipolar disorder is stabilized, treatment for her other challenges can begin. As with residual depression, new medications must be added slowly and carefully to ensure that they do not destabilize her mood. Here are the plus problems most common in children and some of the medications that we use to treat them. We use brand names, but generic products, when available, are usually fine.

### ADHD (ATTENTION DEFICIT HYPERACTIVITY DISORDER, WITH OR WITHOUT HYPERACTIVITY)

- Stimulants, including methylphenidate (Ritalin LA, Concerta), Adderall XR, Adderall IR, Metadate CD, Metadate ER, Dexedrine IR, Dexedrine Spansules, Focalin XR and Focalin, Daytrana (a methylphenidate patch), and Vyvanse

- Nonstimulants, including Strattera. Some other nonstimulants may be helpful for ADHD but don't have FDA approval for this use. These include Provigil (modafinil), Wellbutrin (bupropion), Tenex (guanfacine), clonidine, and tricyclic antidepressants

## ANXIETY (INCLUDING OBSESSIVE-COMPULSIVE DISORDER)

- Selective serotonin reuptake inhibitors (SSRIs), including Prozac, Paxil, Zoloft, Celexa, Luvox, and Lexapro

- Benzodiazepines, including Valium, Ativan, Xanax, Serax, Klonopin, Tranxene, and others

- Selective norepinephrine reuptake inhibitors (SNRIs), including Effexor, Effexor XR, and Cymbalta

- Serzone, BuSpar, and Anafranil

- Anticonvulsants, including valproate, gabapentin, topiramate, and tiagabine

- Adrenergic blockers, including propranolol

## CONDUCT DISORDER AND OPPOSITIONAL DEFIANT DISORDER

- No medical treatment, but the symptoms of these disorders are often fueled by bipolar disorder and ADHD. When bipolar disorder and ADHD are treated, the conduct and oppositional defiant disorders may improve or disappear.

## POLYPHARMACY OR COMBINED PHARMACOTHERAPY

Pharmacotherapy? Polypharmacy? What a mouthful! These terms just mean using drugs to treat a disorder. *Pharmacotherapy* means treatment using medications. *Combined pharmacotherapy* and *polypharmacy* both mean using more than one drug for treatment. Most adults and kids with bipolar take more than one medication to manage their illness. In rare but severe cases, some take as many as a dozen different medications. This can be disconcerting to people who aren't familiar with bipolar treatment, and they may worry that the child is being overmedicated. But in many cases, polypharmacy is appropriate and necessary for effective treatment.

Using multiple medications to treat your child's disorder requires a solid understanding of how each medication acts on its own and how it interacts with the other medications. Your clinician has to evaluate these actions and interactions to determine how they affect the symptoms of bipolar, bipolar plus, and side effects in your child.

## OTHER MEDICAL THERAPIES

### ELECTROCONVULSIVE THERAPY

Electroconvulsive therapy (ECT) is used to treat severe depression, especially if the depression has not responded to treatment with medication. ECT is also sometimes used to treat mania and schizophrenia.

Popular media like to portray ECT as a scary treatment of questionable value, but in its modern forms this treatment has been shown to be safe and effective for adults suffering from severe depression, especially in cases that include psychotic symptoms. ECT can literally be a lifesaver in these situations.

Because no controlled studies using ECT in children or teens have been done, we use it only if other, better-studied options have been unsuccessful. Children ten years old and older have been treated successfully with ECT. Like the antipsychotic medication Clozaril, ECT is considered a treatment of last resort, to be used only if symptoms resist other treatments.

## LIGHT THERAPY

Symptoms of depression in some people occur or worsen in the fall, winter, or early spring. This type of depression is called *seasonal affective disorder* (SAD), and it is linked to fewer hours of daylight. Children and teens with bipolar disorder may also experience this kind of seasonal variation.

During treatment, the person is exposed to bright, full-spectrum light in the early hours of each day to mimic the longer days of summer.

There is a risk that light therapy, just like antidepressant medication, will trigger mania or hypomania in someone who has bipolar, so its use must be monitored carefully.

## TRANSCRANIAL MAGNETICAL STIMULATION

Transcranial magnetical stimulation (TMS) and repeated TMS (r-TMS) are new treatments that are gaining recognition for treating depression, schizophrenia, and obsessive-compulsive disorder. TMS targets a specific area of the brain with a magnetic field, which causes the neurons in that area to fire. Unlike ECT, it does not send an electrical current through the brain and it doesn't trigger a response throughout the brain: It only affects the selected area. Research on the use of TMS to treat mood disorders, including bipolar disorder, has just begun for all age groups. It's too soon to tell whether this will be a safe and effective treatment for bipolar disorder.

## NONPRESCRIPTION
## COMPLEMENTARY TREATMENTS

Recently, several dietary supplements have received attention as possible treatments for depression and other mood disorders. Two of them, essential fatty acids (especially omega-3 fatty acids) and Saint John's wort, have some research supporting their use in adults. Several intriguing case results have been reported for a high-dose nutritional supplement, but no research studies have been completed on it yet.

The use of these options (with or without other medications) has not been extensively studied in the treatment of bipolar disorder, and there is even less research and clinical experience concerning their use in children and teens. Use them with caution and only under careful medical supervision. Do not discontinue known useful medications in favor of complementary treatments without first discussing this with your clinician.

### ESSENTIAL FATTY ACIDS, INCLUDING OMEGA-3

Essential fatty acids are necessary for growth and development, but our bodies don't manufacture them. They enter our system through foods we eat (walnuts; cold-water fish, such as tuna, herring, and salmon; soybeans; leafy greens) or supplements. A diet without enough essential fatty acids can lead to a variety of problems, including changes in how our immune systems, hearts, and brains work.

Some early studies suggest that essential fatty acids, especially omega-3, may alleviate the symptoms of depression and bipolar disorder in adults. Several large studies are under way to explore whether omega-3 fatty acids offer a safe and effective treatment for these illnesses.

At the present time, omega-3 fatty acids may be useful as an adjunctive treatment in adults—not being used *instead* of the usual medications, but as an *additional* treatment that improves overall response to medication. These fatty acids may be similarly useful for children and teens.

In our clinics, we've seen a range of responses to omega-3s. We initially treated Mattie, a five-year-old with mild bipolar symptoms and a strong family history of bipolar disorder, with only omega-3 fatty acids. The omega-3s helped control her symptoms for two years, when she needed to begin taking an atypical antipsychotic. For Tyler, age nine, and Christopher, age fifteen, adding omega-3 fatty acids to their treatment regimen helped decrease residual irritability without their having to take a higher dose of their mood stabilizers. Ten-year-old Heather had better overall mood stability when she took omega-3s; for Debbie, another ten-year-old who was taking the same medications as Heather, omega-3s didn't make a difference. And in at least one case, Astrid, age thirteen, became manic while taking the same form of omega-3s that helped the others.

As with any medication or supplement, essential fatty acids should be taken carefully ("start low and go slow"), under the supervision of your clinician.

### SAINT JOHN'S WORT

Saint John's wort is an herb that may alleviate mild to moderate depression. Research results are mixed. Some (but not all) studies have shown it to be effective for treating mild or moderate depression in adults, but it does not seem to be effective for treating severe depression. There's scant research about its effect on pediatric depression and none on bipolar depression in children or adults.

Because we know so little about the impact of Saint John's wort on bipolar disorder, this herb should be administered with extreme caution and only under your doctor's supervision due to the risk of triggering mania.

Saint John's wort interacts with many other medications, often decreasing their effectiveness. Stopping Saint John's wort abruptly or administering it irregularly can result in withdrawal symptoms, which may be confused with an increase in psychiatric symptoms.

## NUTRITIONAL SUPPLEMENTS

Several case reports regarding a broad-spectrum nutritional supplement suggest that with high doses of the supplement, it's possible to decrease the number and dosages of other medications used to treat bipolar disorder. We don't know yet whether the supplement interacts with other medications or what its long-term impacts and effective dose ranges are. Controlled research studies have not been done.

As with any treatment for bipolar disorder, work with your treatment team to assess whether this approach is appropriate and effective for your child.

---

### NATURAL AND ORGANIC VERSUS SAFE AND EFFECTIVE

If the label says "natural" or "organic," does that mean it's safe to use?

*No.*

Poisonous mushrooms and cyanide are natural, but you wouldn't want to eat them. Cow dung is organic, but it's not good food, either.

Many over-the-counter supplements are not regulated by the FDA. The ingredients in these supplements can (and do) vary by type, purity, and quantity, among other things. In addition, even if a supplement is manufactured by a reliable company that makes sure the product is consistent from batch to batch and contains exactly what the label says, we do not know how the supplement will interact with other medications (or other supplements, for that matter). We have seen people become psychotic after taking a mix of "natural" supplements, so don't risk it. Check with your clinician and your treatment team first.

## NAVIGATING THE TWISTS AND TURNS

There are many medications and treatment options. You know from Figure 4 (page 150) that after being diagnosed with bipolar disorder, your daughter will begin with a trial of a particular medication to see if it helps. If it doesn't, you'll have to try a different medication for her. If it helps but not enough or helps but causes too many side effects, you'll have to change the dose, try a different medication, or add another medication, all, of course, under your clinician's supervision.

How does your doctor know which drug to try first? Where do you and your treatment team begin?

You begin with your child.

In Chapters 2 and 3, you explored the part of the maze that identified symptoms of bipolar and bipolar plus. In Chapter 5, you began using tracking tools to identify your child's symptoms. That's because before beginning treatment and throughout treatment, your doctor needs to know:

• What are your child's symptoms?

• How severe are those symptoms?

This includes information about when and where the symptoms appear (at home, at school, in certain social situations); what triggers the symptoms; how long the symptoms last;

whether the symptoms impair your child's life and development; and how the symptoms affect your child's relationships with other members of your family, and with peers, teachers, teammates, and others.

But that's not all your doctor needs to know. Other factors are important, too:

- How old is your child?

- Has he or she reached puberty?

- Is your child overweight, underweight, or average?

- What else is going on? Bipolar plus? Other medical concerns?

- Is there substance abuse?

- Is there a family history of brain disorders, like bipolar disorder, depression, or alcoholism?

- Is there a family history of other illnesses, like heart disease or diabetes?

- Is there a family history of how family members have responded to medication? A history of the response your child has had to any medications? (The more details, the better.)

- Does your child have any underlying medical problems?

- Is there a family history of serious medical problems?

At first glance, these details may seem unrelated to bipolar. Why does your child's clinician need to know about them?

Because we're not treating just the bipolar disorder, we're treating the whole child.

To do that most effectively, your son's clinician first identifies the options for treating the type and severity of his symptoms. Next, the clinician narrows the options by looking at the potential side effects and possible interactions to determine which medications are most likely to work and least likely to cause serious side effects for him. This winnowing down of options to the one you'll try first is based on the information you've provided. For example, the choices of medication for your son might come down to one of three mood stabilizers. Your doctor might decide to try the one that will likely work the fastest, because of how severe your son's symptoms are; or a different one because there's a history of diabetes in your family; or the third one because of how your son reacted to another medication last year.

Remember, each person reacts to medications differently. Research, clinical experience, and your input guide your clinician to recommend one medication over another, but you and your doctor won't know if it's the right one—the one that is most effective with the fewest side effects—until your son tries it.

Remember, too, that your son's brain is a wonderful and complex organ. Bipolar disorder and the conditions that often accompany it are complicated. It will take time to identify the best match between him and the medications.

## FAMILIES TRAVELING THE
## TREATMENT TWISTS AND TURNS

In this section, we'll travel through the treatment twists and turns with families who've been there. Each story begins with an introduction to the child and a list of major symptoms. Then we examine background information, plus the where, how, and why of the unique path these families are traveling.

These stories are all taken from real people—children and teens with bipolar disorder and their families. Names and personal information have been changed to protect confidentiality; symptoms, treatment details, and reactions to treatment are recounted as they were experienced.

Janey bounded from one side of the examining room to the other. Her bright T-shirt, the patches on the knees of her jeans, even her hair, which refused to stay in its ponytail, reinforced the impression that this eight-year-old was a girl on the go.

- Major temper tantrums, huge scenes, throws and breaks things

- Often extremely happy and excited right before an outburst

- Sleeps a lot less than the typical eight-year-old (and is sleeping less and less)

- Very demanding of Mom; loud and bossy around other kids

- Hyperactive, impulsive

- No friends

Janey's mother says she's always been a "high-maintenance" kid. Janey's parents adopted her when she was an infant. From the beginning, she was "super-active and always on the go." She had a hard time playing on her own, but she tended to alienate other kids because she was bossy. About the time her age-mates were outgrowing this kind of behavior, Janey got much noisier and more destructive.

She began to have mood swings and major temper tantrums. Before an outburst, she appeared wildly excited and happy, but her mother noted that these ebullient moods felt fragile. If whatever followed didn't exactly meet Janey's hopes and expectations, Janey would immediately cause a horrible scene, full of rage. One time when Janey received a gift, she was ecstatic. She opened the gift and discovered a beautiful and hoped-for doll. But because the doll didn't have a second pair of shoes, Janey erupted in a rage storm that lasted for more than half an hour.

Janey sleeps less than is typical for her age, and she has been having increasing difficulty sleeping. She constantly badgers her mom for new things. Other kids avoid her because she is loud and pushy and often gets incredibly angry with them.

Janey's mom works as an aide in the school system and has some experience with special needs children. She says she's always had a sense that ADHD was part of Janey's difficulty, but the rages and angry scenes that are becoming increasingly apparent don't match what she knows about ADHD. She checked into the medical history of Janey's biological family, and there's no record of unusual problems or mental illness. When we completed our evaluation, we agreed that Janey's primary diagnosis was bipolar disorder. She also seems to have ADHD, but we wouldn't know if she needed a medication for that until we stabilized her bipolar.

Because Janey is physically healthy, of normal weight, and has no family history of diabetes, we decided to begin her treatment with Risperdal, an atypical antipsychotic.

She began taking Risperdal (0.5 milligram each day) on October 6. By October 24, just over two weeks later, *all* of her rage and irritability were gone.

Janey is one of a group of children who have a remarkable response to Risperdal. Not all kids respond to atypical antipsychotics, but when they do, we often see improvement within the first three to four weeks of treatment, and sometimes sooner. Rapid response is one of the main reasons that we frequently try atypical antipsychotics first.

At this point, Janey's mother reported that Janey still had ADHD symptoms but they were much easier to handle. Janey was also feeling anxious. This was a problem she had before, but the anxiety seemed to be surfacing a little more since her treatment began.

We considered changing from Risperdal to Seroquel, another atypical antipsychotic, because we thought it might be better for her anxiety. However, Janey's mother said that her response to Risperdal has been so phenomenal that she (and we) didn't want to change medications. Janey's anxiety was manageable and didn't interfere with her regular activities. We discussed the possibility of adding a second medication, Strattera, to address Janey's anxiety and residual ADHD, but decided to wait.

The next step was to monitor Janey's symptoms and how well she was doing until her next office visit in two weeks. If her anxiety increased and began to interfere with her ability to function in social settings during the two weeks, we would look at adjusting the medication right away, before her next appointment. If her anxiety and other symptoms remained stable or continued to improve, we would keep her on Risperdal until we saw her again. Whether we adjusted or changed her medication then would depend on the symptoms her mother observed as well as feedback from Janey herself.

Three weeks into treatment, Janey's bipolar disorder symptoms, primarily rage and irritability, were responding well to Risperdal, and she was tolerating the medicine well. She did not have any residual depression (though this is always a possibility, so we watch for it), and we thought she might still need treatment for anxiety and ADHD. There was also a greater than average chance that Janey had learning disabilities. As her treatment progressed and her symptoms continued to improve, Janey's parents and teachers would be able to more easily identify those learning disabilities and provide appropriate educational support for her.


With his hair combed and his light blue shirt tucked neatly into his dark slacks, Kurt looked like a typical kid from a well-to-do family—if you didn't count his facial expressions. He sneered, glowered, and glared at us with an anger and arrogance far beyond a normal eleven-year-old's.

- Initially he was diagnosed with depression; now he is surly, aggressive, and unruly

- Shoplifting

- Rages; physical fights with his father; throwing furniture; destructive

Kurt's first dramatic mood change happened the summer he was ten. In the spring, his much-beloved grandfather had passed away. Not long after this, Kurt's dog, who had been his constant companion for many years, also died. Because Kurt's grief was severe and unrelenting, his parents took him to their family physician.

The physician diagnosed Kurt with depression triggered by the recent deaths and prescribed the antidepressant Zoloft, one of the selective serotonin reuptake inhibitors, or SSRIs.

By the time Kurt entered middle school that fall, he was angry, unruly, and aggressive. He despised anyone in authority and was convinced that he was superior to everyone. He began shoplifting CDs. He exploded with rage and got into frequent fistfights with his father. He threw furniture and broke anything that was breakable.

Before his grandfather's death, Kurt had been a "good kid"—generally cheerful and helpful, an excellent student, sometimes high-spirited, with above-average intelligence and plenty of creativity. He was sailing smoothly toward a future at the Ivy League college his father had attended. Now it looked like he was developing a serious conduct disorder and heading straight for a life of violence and crime.

When we first met Kurt, the atypical antipsychotic Risperdal was brand-new. Kurt's parents were worried about one of Risperdal's potential side effects, tardive dyskinesia (TD). TD is a movement disorder that develops in some patients after long-term treatment with antipsychotics. It is more likely to occur in patients taking older, first-generation antipsychotics, like Haldol, than with the newer atypical antipsychotics. Time has shown that TD is extremely rare with atypical antipsychotics such as Risperdal, but since the drug was new when Kurt's treatment was first being formulated, and since TD is a risk with any antipsychotic medication, we decided to begin treatment with lithium, the traditional first-line medication for bipolar disorder in adults. Also, because Zoloft had clearly triggered his mania (rages and other aggressive behavior), we decreased and then stopped the Zoloft.

The lithium did not affect Kurt's symptoms. He was still erupting in rage, getting into fights, and shoplifting. Over the next several months, we tried Depakote (valproate, an anticonvulsant), Ativan (lorazepam, a benzodiazepine), and several antianxiety medications.

Kurt's symptoms continued to escalate. They finally became serious enough for us to propose hospitalizing him, for he seemed to be a danger to himself and others. As a last attempt at outpatient treatment, Kurt's parents decided to let us try Risperdal.

Two weeks later, Kurt walked into our office and announced, "Finally, you've given me something that makes me feel better."

Within the next month, Kurt was looking back with horror on his rages and shoplifting. He said he remembered that he had felt invulnerable and believed he was far too clever to be caught. He was appalled at his behavior and aware of how close he'd come to ending up with a criminal record. Kurt's budding conduct disorder completely evaporated as his bipolar disorder was treated. It has never resurfaced.

Risperdal alone did not stabilize his illness, however. Although Kurt's rage decreased, he continued to have many other symptoms and a lot of trouble functioning normally at home and at school. Fourteen years after Kurt's first visit, he takes six medications: Risperdal, Lamictal (an anticonvulsant), and lithium for his bipolar disorder; and Zoloft (yes, Zoloft), BuSpar (an atypical antianxiety medication), and Klonopin (a benzodiazepine) for anxiety.

In addition to taking his medication, Kurt is in daily phone contact with his parents, has a weekly therapy session, and goes for a monthly meds check. He's in a long-term relationship, which has been good for him. His girlfriend has lots of patience and understanding.

He's in college, though not a high-pressure Ivy League school. He earns As and Bs and still performs erratically from time to time, because even though his illness is stable, symptoms break through periodically. Grandiosity crops up— he thinks his teachers are idiots and so refuses to do the coursework—or anxiety flares, paralyzing him with the belief that he's contracted a fatal disease like AIDS.

He takes a lighter course load than he would if he didn't have bipolar disorder. Fewer courses means less stress, which helps him manage his illness. Fewer courses also means fewer pieces to pick up and put back together when symptoms disrupt his ability to function. He is making his way through college, although at a slower pace than many other students.

Kurt's symptom breakthroughs last anywhere from a few days to a few weeks. Sometimes he just rides them out; other times, we increase his Risperdal or lithium dosage.

He's finally learned that regular sleep, exercise, diet, and study habits help him manage his moods better. He's discovered that "recreational" drug use and alcohol can cause major problems—their effects are much worse for him than for others who don't have this illness. He knows that as he graduates from college and begins the next phase of his life, he must continue long-term management of this chronic illness.

Tashina's flair for the dramatic was obvious the first time we saw her. This bright-eyed eleven-year-old bubbled over with energy, dancing around the room, her multicolored skirt swirling, while she told stories in a rapid-fire voice.

- Impulsive, distractible, high-energy, talkative, "spirited," disorganized

- Unexpected reactions to ADHD medications (crying, irritability, argumentativeness, and mood fluctuations)

- Unexpected reactions to antidepressants combined with ADHD medications (screaming, explosive temper tantrums lasting thirty minutes or more every day; bossy and controlling in social situations; trashes any room she's playing in)

- Biting, kicking, hitting; threw and broke things

- Told "tall tales," exaggerated popularity

- No longer modest about being naked in the house

- Flagrant disregard for all authority; refused to do schoolwork or anything parents requested

- Poor school performance despite high intelligence and imagination

- Slept about the same amount as other kids her age

- Slightly overweight

By the time Tashina was eight, everybody agreed that she had ADHD. She was bright and imaginative; she was also impulsive, distractible, and disorganized. In preschool, one optimistic teacher had labeled her a "spirited kid"—a nice way of saying she talked nonstop and had more energy than she knew what to do with.

In third grade, her school suggested that she be evaluated. Her diagnosis was ADHD and she began taking Ritalin (methylphenidate); soon she was switched to Concerta, another form of methylphenidate in which the drug is released at a constant rate over an eight- to twelve-hour period. She started to cry a lot more, so her doctor changed her medication to Adderall, another stimulant frequently used to treat ADHD. At first, Tashina seemed calmer and could think better, but then, about six weeks after switching to Adderall, she had a flare-up of irritability, argumentativeness, and mood fluctuations. By late summer, it was clear that Tashina had a mood disorder. In November, her doctor started her on Paxil, a commonly used SSRI antidepressant. She had fewer meltdowns and seemed much improved. Then her doctor increased the dosage of both Adderall and Paxil to treat "residual symptoms."

By February, Tashina was erupting in one or two violent, screaming tantrums every day. Each tantrum lasted half an hour or more. When she wasn't throwing a tantrum, Tashina was bossy and controlling, alienating her friends. Her mother said Tashina "played as if a tornado had gone through"—she pulled out all her toys, put none of them away, played with everything but couldn't settle on any one thing, and completely trashed the room.

Tashina's meds were slowly decreased and then stopped, but she continued to do poorly. She had the full range of

ADHD symptoms plus violent and destructive outbursts that included hitting, kicking, and biting. She began to tell tall tales, especially ones that exaggerated her popularity. She had been reasonably modest about nudity; now she didn't care if she was naked anywhere in the house. She defied anyone in authority and refused to do homework or anything her parents asked her to.

At this point, Tashina's parents brought her to our clinic. Because Tashina was a little overweight, we decided to treat her with Abilify instead of another atypical antipsychotic, such as Risperdal or Zyprexa. These are all likely to produce a quick response, but one of the common side effects of both Risperdal and Zyprexa is weight gain (an average of five pounds in eight weeks for Risperdal and twice that for Zyprexa). Abilify does not have that particular side effect in most people.

Soon after Tashina began taking Abilify, her mother called. Tashina loved drama and performing onstage—drama was the one activity she'd been able to do no matter how bad her symptoms were—but that night, during a dress rehearsal in front of a small audience, she had refused to go onstage. She was crying and complained of a stomachache. At first, they thought she was sick, but she recovered soon after they got home. If taking Abilify meant she would experience a panic attack every time she tried to perform, then the medication wasn't the right one for her.

Because Tashina had had poor results and bad side effects from so many medications in less than a year, her parents decided to wait before trying anything new. They agreed to track Tashina's moods and behavior and to touch base with us by phone at least once a month.

After three months with no medication, her parents reported to us that Tashina was having huge reactions to tiny triggers. When she didn't get the seat that she wanted in the car, she screamed, cried, and refused to get into the car. She had nighttime energy surges, with giddy, goofy behavior and manic laughter. She often seemed to be filled with bouncy energy and was even more of a chatterbox than she was before. Irritability flared up at unpredictable moments. Every minute of her day had to be filled with social contact.

Clearly, we all agreed, it was time to try medication again. There were many choices that had not yet been tried with Tashina, and somewhere in that collection lay a prescription for real relief for her—and her family, friends, and school.

This time, Tashina began taking 1 milligram of Risperdal at bedtime. After two months, she had gained some weight, which was a problem, and she was a bit lethargic. Of greater concern were her mood swings. They weren't as severe as they had been, but she continued to have angry spells during which she lashed out for brief periods, giddy spells that were mostly annoying, and anxiety, when she would question her capacity to do things. In addition, Tashina, who had always been smart enough to get through her classes with As and Bs, was getting Cs in everything. It was clear that she wasn't living up to her academic expectations, which reinforced her anxiety. It was time for an adjustment in her medication.

We lowered her Risperdal to .75 milligram to reduce the side effects and added Strattera (a selective norepinephrine reuptake inhibitor, or SNRI) to help with ADHD and anxiety. This treatment regimen was much more successful.

Tashina finished the school year with four As, one B, and a C; she said that only her reading class was hard. Since then, her grades have been As and Bs. She likes science and math but rushes through the work, missing important details—an ADHD-type symptom—but does well enough to get Bs anyway. She still needs plenty of social interaction and lots of activities, and she has friends who like and value her.

She's no longer physically aggressive, although she can be mean-spirited, especially to her siblings. For the time being, Tashina's mother is using a behavioral approach to deal with this: Every time Tashina gets caught being nasty to a sibling, she must do something nice for that person. Her moods are still changeable—she'll go from grouchy to happy to upset in the blink of an eye—but her volatility is much less intense. Her teacher reports that Tashina handles school well for the most part, though by the end of the day, Tashina often exhibits pressured speech or an increase in chattiness.

At the lower level of Risperdal, Tashina's weight is stable and she isn't lethargic. She is, however, having difficulty getting enough sleep. She falls asleep so late that she's hard to rouse in the morning. Her schoolwork, ADHD symptoms, and mood might all improve with better sleep.

Sleep hygiene is an important part of good management of bipolar, and it can be a major challenge. The internal clocks of people with bipolar disorder are often askew, and their brains, like Tashina's, want to be awake late into the night. Adding to the challenge is that bad or manic moods can disrupt sleep, and sleep deprivation can trigger bad or manic moods.

To help Tashina improve her sleep, she has begun taking Seroquel in addition to Risperdal at bedtime. Seroquel is another atypical antipsychotic; mild sedation is one of its more common side effects. Adding Seroquel was preferable to increasing her Risperdal dose, since we already knew that for Tashina higher levels of Risperdal would cause weight gain and lethargy, giving her too much sedation during the day.

Depending on how Tashina responds to the Seroquel, we might want to increase her Strattera dose in the future.

Lonnie was skinny and tall for a ten-year-old. She wore a dark purple leotard with butterflies silk-screened on the front, a short denim skirt, and purple tights.

- Erratic mood cycles

- Hypersexuality

- Drug and alcohol abuse

- Suicide threats and attempts

We first met Lonnie when she was ten years old. She committed suicide ten years later, when she was twenty.

We include her story for two important reasons. First, it serves as a reminder that bipolar disorder is a challenging chronic illness, often difficult to treat and fraught with peril. Kids with bipolar disorder are kids at risk—for drug and alcohol abuse, for dangerous behavior that shows up when mania breaks through, for suicide.

Second, Lonnie's story illustrates the dangers of stopping medication abruptly, whether by the patient's choice or for other medical reasons, as was the case with Lonnie.

Lonnie had already been diagnosed with ADHD when she came to see us. She'd had an allergic skin reaction to Tegretol (an anticonvulsant) and got grouchier when she tried Tenex (a medication for high blood pressure that is also used to treat ADHD). She'd tried the stimulant Ritalin, frequently used to treat ADHD, but it didn't help much and she developed a tic. She was currently taking clonidine (a nonstimulant ADHD medication) and Dexedrine (a stimulant).

To her ADHD diagnosis, we added the diagnoses of bipolar disorder, plus panic disorder, social phobia, and generalized anxiety disorder. We prescribed lithium and Risperdal to treat Lonnie's bipolar disorder, continued the Dexedrine for ADHD, and gradually phased out the clonidine. Two months later, we added Paxil (an SSRI) to treat her anxiety and depression, but her mood swings increased dramatically, so we decreased the Paxil and added nortriptyline (a tricyclic antidepressant).

Four months later, Lonnie was suicidal and refused to go to school. The lithium wasn't helping her symptoms, and its side effects—increased thirst and bloating—were uncomfortable enough that she stopped taking the medication. We tried Klonopin (a benzodiazepine) and Zoloft (a different SSRI) for anxiety, increased her Risperdal, and switched her to a different form of Dexedrine.

Over the next ten years, Lonnie's meds changed regularly as her symptoms flared and shifted. Always, our starting point in treating her was to address the symptoms of bipolar disorder. We also changed and adjusted her medications to treat her sleep problems, anxiety, depression, eating disorder, cocaine use—and the side effects from her various medications.

In her early teens, Lonnie began to have serious problems with hypersexuality. She developed indiscriminate sexual behaviors and began to drink alcohol and smoke marijuana.

These behaviors, which were driven by her illness, put her in dangerous situations. Once, she ended up wearing nothing but lingerie in an isolated park late at night, accompanied by several older teen boys, who claimed they were making a movie. A few months later, she left unannounced for another city to meet in person a man she'd connected with online. She thought he was her age but discovered that he was in his fifties. She managed to call her mother for help. Her mother contacted the local police, who got her back home.

Her moods ran through cycles that varied every day. One moment she was loud and shouting in the rapid-fire pressured speech common in mania, demanding to buy clothes and makeup while planning for her big career as a model and actress. The next moment, she'd be threatening suicide.

Even with meds, outpatient therapy, and her parents' love and close supervision, Lonnie's life was chaotic and dangerous, so when she was sixteen, she began attending a therapeutic boarding school. This high school helped keep her safe by providing around-the-clock supervision and structure as well as emotional and academic support.

At nineteen, she moved to a less restrictive (although still supervised) environment, and then she tried college. She was relatively stable on a combination of Lamictal (an anticonvulsant), Abilify and Seroquel (both atypical antipsychotics), and Klonopin (a benzodiazepine).

College began well, but by the end of her first semester, Lonnie's symptoms were worsening. She wasn't able to keep up with class requirements and was becoming increasingly anxious. In January, she complained that her meds kept "wearing off" and admitted that she was using cocaine. She refused to take several of her meds. Lonnie continued to use cocaine through the spring; she tried to stop several times but relapsed.

In April, Lonnie almost succeeded in committing suicide by taking an entire bottle of Tylenol (acetaminophen). This caused serious damage to her liver and for a time it looked like she would survive only with a liver transplant. Eventually, she recovered enough liver function to avoid the transplant but not enough to continue taking her medications as before.

After this suicide attempt, Lonnie left college and moved home to live with her parents. Within weeks, she had fallen head-over-heels in love and was planning her wedding. Her new boyfriend, initially as enthusiastic and smitten as she was, changed his mind and broke up with her. Two weeks later, after many emotional phone calls with him, Lonnie took her own life.

Suicide was always a significant risk for Lonnie; threats and attempts had been part of her bipolar disorder from the beginning. When her medication was stopped abruptly because of the liver damage from her suicide attempt at college, her risk of suicide and other symptoms of bipolar disorder escalated. The liver damage from her Tylenol overdose required us to significantly change the amounts and types of medications she took, making her bipolar disorder even more challenging for us and her parents to control.

In the end, even the love and support of Lonnie's family, her ongoing medical treatment, and therapy were not enough to overcome the severe symptoms of her illness.

## THE DANGER OF SUICIDE

People, including teens and young children, with bipolar disorder have an increased risk of suicide, even when their illness is being treated. If someone you know talks about, threatens, or attempts suicide, take it seriously!

*If you or someone you know is feeling suicidal or is in crisis and you need help right away:*
Call 911, your doctor, or the hospital emergency room.
Call the National Suicide Prevention Lifeline:
1-800-273-TALK (1-800-273-8255).
They're available twenty-four hours a day, seven days a week. All calls are confidential.
*Para obtener asistencia en español:* 1-888-628-9454.
Make sure that the suicidal person is not left alone, and that anything that could be used for self-harm—medications or weapons, for example—is inaccessible.

*Signs and symptoms that may accompany suicidal feelings include:*
• Talking about feeling suicidal or wanting to die
• Feeling hopeless, that nothing will ever change or get better
• Feeling like a burden to family and friends
• Abusing alcohol or drugs
• Putting affairs in order (for example, organizing finances or giving away personal possessions)
• Writing a suicide note
• Putting oneself in harm's way or in situations where there is a danger of being killed

For more information about suicide risk, warning signs, and what to do, see Chapter 11.

Tara clutched her mother's hand and glanced around the room warily as they stepped through the doorway. She clung to her mother the way a shy toddler would, although Tara was a bright, creative, eight-year-old. She was overweight and looked tired.

- Irritable; explosive rages; outbursts occurred many times per day and lasted twenty minutes to two hours

- Exhausted and sad after outbursts

- Hit, punched, spat, threw things when she didn't get her way

- Out of control at home and at school

- Trouble sleeping

- Periods of extreme silliness and uncontrollable laughing

- Hallucinations (ghosts—visual and auditory)

- Lots of anxiety—couldn't be in room alone, was terrified of being separated from her parents

- Family history of bipolar disorder

Tara's days—and nights—were volatile: the spinning star common with early-onset bipolar disorder. She was sometimes sweet and kind, but had frequent severe outbursts at home and at school. Her outbursts could last as long as two hours and left her drained and weepy. Her behavior in the car whenever she didn't get her way endangered everyone—she hit, punched, threw things, kicked the back of her mother's seat, and flung herself to the floor as she screamed and raged. She had trouble sleeping. Her silly moods were giddy and over the top, with uncontrollable laughter. She had hallucinations of ghosts coming at her, sometimes speaking to her. She was extremely anxious. She refused to be in a room by herself and she was terrified of being separated from her parents. She also had a family history of bipolar disorder: Her uncle, who was no longer alive, had been diagnosed as an adult and had been treated with mixed results.

Tara began taking Abilify (an atypical antipsychotic), which helped somewhat, but it did not control her symptoms completely. She also gained weight once she started taking it, even though weight gain isn't typically one of Abilify's side effects. Since the Abilify was partially effective, we decided to keep it at the current level and add another mood stabilizer for the residual symptoms. We ended up adding two medications, one at a time, plus an omega-3 fatty acid supplement.

Each day Tara took Abilify (5 milligrams two times a day), the anticonvulsant Trileptal (150 milligrams three times a day), Lithobid, a slow release form of lithium (300 milligrams twice a day), and four capsules of omega-3 fatty acids.

She tolerated all these medications well and several months later reported that school was "perfect"—two big thumbs-up. She'd been having a little trouble with after-school activities, so we shifted the timing of her second Abilify dose and she did much better.

She still got a little hyper and silly, but settled down quickly. She still got angry and frustrated when she had trouble with her schoolwork or when things didn't go the way she wanted, but she didn't explode into rage storms.

She struggled to make friends but enjoyed playing with other kids. She had one good friend and was part of a lunch group. Her weight was stable, and she was sleeping better, too.

The omega-3 supplement didn't seem to be helping and it was expensive, so the family began tapering it off. One day Tara became agitated and said that she felt "crazy" and very tired. On another day, she missed her afternoon meds and that evening had a panic attack severe enough to require a trip to the emergency room.

Now that Tara's moods were stabilizing, her mother had noticed a lot of ADHD symptoms (inattention, trouble sitting and listening, and hyperactivity but not mania). Tara wasn't as sad lately, her mother reported, but she was impulsive, would get fixated or hyperfocused on certain things, and was still easily frustrated and impatient.

Tara had been treated for ADHD when she was four to five years old, before she was diagnosed and treated for bipolar disorder. Concerta made her agitated; Ritalin resulted in insomnia; Strattera didn't do anything; Wellbutrin didn't work and might have made her mood worse; and Adderall did make her mood worse.

We decided to increase her dosage of the anticonvulsant Trileptal to further stabilize her mood before tackling the ADHD symptoms, especially since improved mood might also result in improved ADHD symptoms.

Tara's mood did stabilize with the increase in Trileptal. Her ADHD symptoms were still causing significant problems, so we carefully and slowly introduced Adderall XR. Unfortunately, the stimulant medication destabilized her mood, and it took several months to regain control of her mood and anxiety symptoms. We decided for the time being to keep her on her current medications, which were effectively treating her bipolar and anxiety disorders, and work with nonmedical supports to help with her ADHD symptoms.

Timothy was a towheaded urchin, three and a half years old, with a grin that could steal your heart—when he wasn't exploding in one of his frequent rages.

- Irritable, cranky, and inconsolable even as an infant

- Frequent, extreme temper tantrums; violent aggression; head-banging when angry

- Hyperactive; impulsive

- Fearless; engaged in dangerous and risky behavior

- Extreme mood swings

- Strong family history of bipolar disorder, including two completed suicides

- Diagnosed with bipolar disorder at three and a half years

Timothy began showing symptoms of a mood disorder as an infant. He was irritable, didn't sleep well, and cried all the time. He wasn't able to bond well with his parents or anyone else. His symptoms got worse as he entered his toddler years: He had severe temper tantrums with biting, screaming, and violent aggression; hyperactivity and impulsivity far beyond that of a normal two- or three-year-old; head-banging when he was angry; dangerous behavior and risk-taking; and, no surprise, extreme mood swings.

Because he has a strong family history of bipolar disorder, including two close relatives who committed suicide, Timothy's parents suspected early on that their son might have this illness. We diagnosed Timothy with bipolar disorder when he was only three and a half years old.

The early onset of Timothy's symptoms—possibly evident shortly after his birth—and his significant family history made it especially important for us to begin treatment as soon as possible.

We began him on Abilify: 2.5 milligrams, twice a day. The medication helped but did not resolve all of Timothy's symptoms. Increasing his Abilify dose made him too sleepy, so we added Depakote (an anticonvulsant; 300 milligrams twice a day). This helped for a while but then stopped working. When we increased the Depakote, his anxiety also increased and his rages became more extreme. So we cross-tapered (decreased one medication while introducing and increasing another) and shifted him from Depakote to Zyprexa (an atypical antipsychotic). That worked well for a time, though he gained a lot of weight on both Abilify and Zyprexa.

After his mood stabilized on Zyprexa, we added Strattera, which helped alleviate Timothy's hyperactivity and impulsivity. Zyprexa eventually stopped working and Timothy's weight increased, so we cross-tapered to Seroquel (another atypical antipsychotic). The combination of Seroquel and Strattera helped him considerably, but he had some insomnia and mild residual irritability. We reintroduced a small amount of Zyprexa, since that was the only thing that had worked for sleep in the past.

For fifteen months, Timothy was stable on 10 milligrams of Strattera in the mornings, 100 milligrams of Seroquel taken twice a day, and 5 milligrams of Zyprexa at bedtime. Then his moods worsened. We edged his Seroquel dose up bit by bit over several weeks to make sure he could tolerate it. When it reached 200 milligrams twice a day, he began doing better again. Because he still had some residual symptoms of mania, we increased his Zyprexa to 5 milligrams twice a day, and his moods once again stabilized.

Jeremy was a tall, lean sixteen-year-old who first visited us when he was a preschooler.

- Irritable, restless, and low-level agitation

- His parents say he's "joyless"; he says he's "bored"

- Favorite activities—video games and memorizing lines from funny movies—no longer hold his interest for any length of time

- Behavior and attitude have become more annoying and more irritating

- Lately, has been saying things like, "I'll never amount to anything," "Everybody hates me," "No wonder nobody likes me"

- Recently moved and is attending a much larger high school

Jeremy was diagnosed with bipolar disorder plus Asperger's syndrome when he was five years old. When he was younger, his main bipolar symptoms were severe rage storms, energized euphoria especially in the evening, and a lot of difficulty getting to sleep. Over the years, he's responded well first to Risperdal and then to Abilify.

His family recently moved and Jeremy is attending a new school. He and his parents recognize that Jeremy is feeling a lot of stress from the noisy hallways and bigger classes, and his parents have begun looking for a smaller school for him to attend. They're also helping him to cultivate social relationships in their new neighborhood. At home, Jeremy is both irritable and irritating. He hasn't erupted in any rage storms, but he is constantly picking on his brother and sister, sometimes literally poking them.

Jeremy is clearly struggling with bipolar depression. We begin his treatment with 25 milligrams Lamictal in the morning, with instructions to increase the dose by 25 milligrams every week, aiming for a final daily dose of 150 milligrams, all taken in the morning (some people have sleep disturbances if they take Lamictal at night). During this time, he'll continue taking his usual dose of Abilify (20 milligrams each morning), too. When he's tapered up to 150 milligrams of Lamictal each day, he'll return for a follow-up appointment.

We emphasized to both Jeremy and his parents that it was extremely important to increase the Lamictal slowly—from starting dose to target dose would take six weeks—because with the slow, gradually increasing taper, Stevens-Johnson syndrome or other serious rashes are exceedingly rare.

The Stevens-Johnson syndrome is Lamictal's most serious potential side effect. Jeremy and his parents need to be alert to skin changes that could be a sign of this allergic rash reaction. Although rare, this rash can be severe, sometimes life-threatening. The most worrisome skin signs to watch out for are blistering around the mouth, palms, or genital areas. If they noticed any skin changes, they should immediately contact their family doctor or, better yet, a dermatologist.

Jeremy and his parents followed the gradual increase instructions and partway into the third week, his parents noticed redness around Jeremy's cheeks and eyes. In their family doctor's office, they realized that Jeremy had been outside a lot that day—it wasn't the beginnings of a Stevens-Johnson rash, it was sunburn. He had a sunburn pattern on his forearms, too, which helped confirm that the redness on his face was sunburn (and that he needed to remember to use sunblock the next time).

They continued the gradual increase up to 150 milligrams and, although things were better, Jeremy still had symptoms of depression, so we tapered up to 200 milligrams over the next two weeks. At the new dose, Jeremy appeared happier, was again interested in his favorite activities, was initiating social interaction on his own instead of waiting for his mom to do that for him, had stopped making negative self-esteem comments, and wasn't bugging his siblings all the time. He's continued to do well on a daily regimen of 200 milligrams Lamictal and 20 milligrams Abilify, both taken once a day in the morning.

The risk of Stevens-Johnson syndrome is extremely rare provided that you begin with a low dose and taper up gradually. It's important to be alert for any skin changes that could signal the beginning of this rash, and we recommend that you contact a dermatologist to examine any change you notice. Dermatologists specialize in skin conditions and can recognize whether something serious is beginning or not. That redness might be from sunburn, poison ivy, acne, or any number of other harmless causes. One of the ones that surprised us recently was contact dermatitis—a rash caused by contact with a substance. Craig, who had been taking Lamictal for several weeks, developed a rash on his arms and face. The dermatologist realized the rash was a reaction from hairspray (he smelled Craig's arm, which still had a faint perfumey smell). Craig explained that his hair had a weird shape to it that morning and he'd tried to mash it in place with his mom's hairspray.

If you notice a skin change, you don't need to panic—but you do need to have a clinician experienced with skin rashes take a look.

Medication is a powerful ally in treating bipolar disorder, and for many kids it will be part of their treatment for their entire life. But even without that lifelong commitment, these cases show how important treatment is in the here-and-now for these kids.

Effective medical treatment of their illness may also open the way for therapy and education. Michael's mother said, "Deciding to give my son meds was one of the hardest things I've ever had to do. It's also turned out to be one of the best decisions I've made. For the first time in a long time, he's able to participate, to learn. It's as if the bipolar was a castle wall and the meds opened the door to let the love and lessons of family, school, and therapy in."

Bipolar disorder is a chronic illness that requires long-term management, including treatment plans like those discussed in this chapter, but it takes more than medication to treat a child affected by bipolar disorder. In the next chapter, we'll take a look at types of therapies that can help you and your family.

*Chapter 8*

# DOORS AND DETOURS

## FINDING PSYCHOTHERAPY THAT HELPS

*I like it and I don't like it, mostly because of having something that makes me different. I get confident of my ideas being able to work, and it's super-clear how to do video games. Bipolar gives me a smiley feeling. That feeling is usually hard for me. What's bad about it is that it messes up my logic, like I'm thinking if I get myself in trouble, everyone will be disappointed in themselves and not me. When I'm mad, I need to protect other people, so I make them mad at me. I get sad sometimes; I had to go to the hospital because I overdosed.*

JEREMY, AGE TWELVE, DIAGNOSED AGE SIX

Successful treatment for bipolar disorder involves more than finding the right combination of meds. Like other chronic illnesses, bipolar puts enormous stress on everyone in your child's world, and especially on members of your immediate family: you, your spouse (including ex-spouses and step-parents), and your other children. How you and your family members react to and manage the impact of bipolar depends on many factors—the type and severity of symptoms, the age and maturity of your child, the needs and reactions of siblings, the skills and support you have, and more. Over time, you and your family as well as your child with bipolar may benefit from psychotherapy or other support.

There is no evidence that psychotherapy alone will remedy the core symptoms of bipolar disorder. We do have evidence that certain drugs can help; that's why treatment with medication typically comes first. However, once symptoms are stabilized, various types of therapy can be tremendously helpful. Studies have shown that certain types of therapy can lead to better mood stability, fewer hospitalizations, and better functioning in many areas. Psychotherapy can help kids and their families understand the illness and why meds and other management issues are important. Plus disorders, behavior and learning problems, and substance abuse, all often part of the bipolar picture, need to be addressed, too. A good therapist can help each individual and the family as a whole cope with feelings and symptoms and can facilitate changes in behavior.

Another reason to include therapy as part of treatment is that, often, medication plus therapy works much better than either alone and better than the simple sum of the two. We think the reason for this is because medication and therapy activate different parts of the brain, and there may be feedback between those systems which enhances the results even more.

There are different kinds of therapy, just like there are different kinds of medication. Some focus on problems specific to bipolar disorder; others tackle broader problems such as communication. What works for your child now might be different from what worked a year ago and will almost certainly be different from what you'll need next year or the year after that. Your child might benefit from one type of therapy or from a particular therapist for many years, supplementing this ongoing work with shorter bursts of other programs. Her regular therapy might be suspended while she attends a therapeutic residential school or she might shift to a new therapist when she's in her teens. Brothers and sisters might attend group sessions specially designed for siblings. You might join a parent support group, attend advocacy training, go to counseling on your own, and participate in couples or family therapy, all at different times over the years.

In this chapter, you'll find descriptions of the therapies most often used to help kids who have bipolar and their families. Which one will be best depends on what you, your child, and your family need at any given time. It's impractical and expensive to try all the options at once. With the help of your treatment team, you must identify problem areas and decide which are most important or cause the greatest difficulties. The problem at the top of the list is the one to work on first, using the therapeutic approach best suited for it. For example, if your son is struggling with friendships and social skills, entering him in a therapy group that works on friendships and social skills may be a good choice. If there's a lot of discord in the family, family therapy or collaborative problem solving may be the place to begin. If your daughter is suffering from anxiety or depression, she may benefit from cognitive behavioral therapy (CBT) or dialectical behavior therapy (DBT).

Most therapists use a combination of approaches, and most don't list those approaches on the door out front—and that's okay, because the name of the approach isn't the most important element of therapy. There is room, and need, for all of the types and styles we've included in this chapter, and more besides.

Even when you know it's time to begin psychotherapy, it's not always clear what therapeutic approach or therapist is best. For example, if your marriage is suffering from the strain of your child's problems, you might decide to see a marriage counselor or couples therapist. If the therapist doesn't know anything about kids with bipolar, she may be missing the information that will be most useful to you as the parents. On the other hand, huge difficulties communicating with your spouse might be an entirely separate issue from your kid-with-bipolar issues, and it might not matter if the therapist is inexperienced regarding kids like yours if she's well versed in spouse communication problems.

The first time you talk with a therapist, you need to ask some basic questions, just as you do when you're considering anyone for your treatment team. Both the answers you get and how you feel during the conversation determine whether this particular therapist is the right therapist, right now. Ask:

- What do you offer? What is your basic approach to treatment?

- What is your experience with and knowledge about mood disorders in kids like mine?

- How much will it cost? What are the payment options for costs that aren't covered by my insurance?

- What is your recommended treatment regimen? Some therapeutic approaches are short-term and focus on one or two specific problems. Others are long-term. Some are one-to-one, others are one or two therapists plus one or more family members or a therapist plus a group of unrelated clients. Some are combinations of these. None of them are right or wrong; which one is best depends on what you and your child need. One family we work with has participated in twice-a-week therapy sessions for ten years. It's taken a lot of time and money, but it helped all three kids build judgment skills and was what they needed. Another family didn't need the same thing; they benefited from short-term family therapy with occasional returns to the same therapist for "tune-ups." And just because you start with one regimen or approach doesn't mean you have to stick with it for life. If the therapy isn't helping, try something else. (See "How Do You Know If It's Working?" below.)

The therapies listed below are all supported by research, but as with medications, much more research has been done with adults than children. Researchers continue to explore how different therapeutic methods compare with each other and how they can help kids and their families.

## HOW DO YOU KNOW IF IT'S WORKING?

Therapy—regardless of type—should be helpful!

Sounds obvious, but sometimes that simple goal gets lost in all the hubbub.

What does "helpful" mean?

The specific goals of therapy depend on the needs of the person who's in therapy—you, your child, your entire family—and the type of therapist, but the big, overarching goal is that therapy should result in positive change. "Positive change" means different things to different people, too, but in general, therapy should improve quality of life, prevent or reduce the damage that bipolar can cause to relationships, help build independence and responsibility, and help your child live, grow, and develop as normally as possible.

If the therapist doesn't use one of the categories we've described in this chapter but has a good relationship with you and your child and the therapy seems to be helping, stay with that therapist. If the therapist you've found is using one or more of these techniques but there's no connection or the therapy doesn't seem to be helping, consider finding a different therapist. The type of therapy is important, but so is the "match" between therapist and patient.

## COLLABORATIVE PROBLEM SOLVING

Collaborative problem solving (CPS), developed by Ross W. Greene, helps teach the cognitive skills needed to handle frustration and to master situations that require flexibility and adaptability. CPS specifically addresses challenging behaviors that are disrupting family life, whether or not anyone in the family has a particular psychiatric diagnosis.

The underlying premise of CPS is that kids who erupt in extreme behaviors such as explosive rage or severe withdrawal do so because they don't have the cognitive flexibility and tolerance for frustration that other kids their age have. This difficulty, like a learning disability, could be part of your child's wiring whether or not she has bipolar or any other diagnosis. And, as with a learning disability, it's possible to put some strategies into place to help your child compensate.

Greene divides typical adult responses to a child's explosive behavior into three categories. "Plan A" is when the adult handles a situation by fiat: "It's my way or the highway," as the old saying goes. If your son says he's too tired to do his homework and you say, "Too bad, do it now," you're using Plan A. If your daughter says she wants ice cream for breakfast and you say, "No!" you're using Plan A.

Lots of us grew up in Plan A families, but if you have a kid with bipolar, you already know that Plan A leads to blowups, not compliance, most of the time.

"Plan C" means you're dropping the expectation completely, at least for now. You're not "giving in" or "giving up"; you've simply decided that for the time being, you're not going to expect something you'd normally expect. Sometimes we lump Plan A and Plan C together and call it "picking our battles." If you decide that for today (or for this week) it isn't worth it to risk a rage storm over ice cream for breakfast, you're using Plan C. You're also using Plan C when you lower your expectations across the board because your child's mood isn't stabilized.

"Plan B" is collaborative problem solving (CPS). It has two big advantages over Plans A and C. First, it gives you more options than "big risk of explosion versus ignoring problems." Second, it teaches a step-by-step approach that helps your child learn how to improve his cognitive flexibility and handle frustrations more effectively.

In CPS, you and your child figure out together what the problem is, what the concerns are, and one or more solutions that each of you will try the next time the situation or problem arises. This approach helps your child (and you) think through things when he's frustrated, regardless of why he's frustrated. It helps put options and alternatives in place before he needs them, so he doesn't have to "think fast" at a time when he's emotionally overloaded and struggling to think at all.

The CPS process can help preempt explosions. With consistent, long-term use, many (but not all) kids will develop the capacity to use the process on their own, without needing you to facilitate. Those who don't may benefit from a different type of therapy, for example, interpersonal therapy (IPT).

## INDIVIDUAL AND FAMILY PSYCHOEDUCATIONAL THERAPY

Psychoeducational therapy teaches you, your child, and other family members about your child's illness, from symptoms and their impact on the family to treatment options and relapse prevention. You learn coping strategies and problem-solving skills that enable you to handle the challenges generated by your child's illness more effectively. Your child develops a better understanding of his illness and why meds and other management issues are so important. The education, social support, and skill building all contribute to better symptom management and family functioning.

Psychoeducation is often interwoven with other therapies. The team member who prescribes your son's meds talks to you about the meds, what to expect, and what to watch out for. Routine med-check appointments include ongoing discussions about managing the illness, not just "here's a refill." Family therapists and couples counselors use information about bipolar to put family and marriage difficulties into context, identify patterns that aren't working, and explore new strategies to try.

## COGNITIVE BEHAVIORAL THERAPY

Cognitive behavioral therapy (CBT) incorporates cognitive therapy, which examines how thoughts affect emotions, and behavioral therapy, which works to help the client change his response to challenging situations. The idea behind CBT is that what we believe about a situation affects how we feel about the situation, and how we feel determines how we behave.

In CBT, the therapist helps you or your child or other family member identify thoughts that are irrational, distorted, inaccurate, or simply not helpful, and what specifically about those thoughts is causing problems. Next, you work on becoming aware of those thoughts, challenging or rejecting them when they occur, and replacing them with more realistic, useful thoughts. Research studies have shown that CBT combined with medication can help kids with bipolar reduce the severity of their mood swings and may help prevent, delay, or reduce the severity of relapses or symptom breakthroughs.

The first part of the CBT process—identifying problem thoughts and why they're a problem—involves three steps first described by Albert Ellis as the "ABCs of Irrational Beliefs."

> *A* is the "activating" event or situation; something happens.
> *B* is "belief." You believe or think something about the situation.
> *C* is "consequences." You have an emotional reaction to the belief and behaviors that stem from that belief.

The activating situation doesn't cause your emotional reaction and behavior; your belief about the situation does. If you believed something else about the situation, you'd have a different emotional reaction, which would lead to different behavior.

Imagine you've walked into the lobby of an elegant hotel and everyone turns to look at you. Why do you think they're staring? Is it because you're a low-class nobody? Or because you're positively glamorous? Or do you believe that the staring has nothing to do with you at all? How you feel will depend on what you believe to be true about the situation; the situation itself is the same regardless of what you believe.

The second part of CBT—challenging problem beliefs and replacing them with more accurate, rational, and helpful ones—involves time, effort, and practice. Here's an example.

Medication has helped stabilize Eric's moods, but he still has what his mom calls "hot spots"—situations that are likely to trigger severe rage storms. Grocery stores are especially challenging. Impulsivity, irritability, and "mission mode" make an explosive combination.

Eric and his family use several techniques to cope with the situation, including avoiding grocery stores as much as possible. Eric knows that grocery stores are a trigger, though he doesn't always know why. When he sees something in the store that he wants, his first thought is, "I have to have it now."

As part of his CBT, Eric has begun to practice "self-talk" that helps him recognize this thought as one he wants to replace. He is also practicing several "replacement" thoughts, "I want it and I can wait," and "I already decided that I want ice cream at the park, not a candy bar here in the store," for example.

CBT helps us look at situations in different ways. Therapists call this "reframing"; you might think of it as looking at the situation from a different angle. Lots of people reframe naturally without ever being aware of it. It may not be until you're tackling the challenges of a kid with bipolar that you discover some problem thoughts of your own. CBT can help here, too.

Nathan and his dad fought constantly. Nathan was defiant, oppositional, and confrontational. His dad was angry and frustrated. "If I'd acted like that when I was a kid, my old man would've thrashed me," he fumed.

Nathan's dad analyzed his thoughts about these confrontations. He realized that his underlying belief was that any kid who acted the way Nathan did was deliberately challenging his authority and would only shape up if Dad laid down the law.

But Nathan's behavior wasn't willful; it was a direct result of his illness. In addition, Nathan's oppositional behavior—like that of many kids with bipolar—got worse in response to authority. The more heavy-handed the authority, the more severe the oppositional behavior.

Nathan's dad switched tactics. Instead of interpreting these situations as threats to his authority, he reframed them as symptoms of Nathan's illness. Now he could focus on helping Nathan, instead of engaging him in an escalating power struggle.

## DIALECTICAL BEHAVIOR THERAPY

Dialectical behavior therapy (DBT), developed by Marsha M. Linehan, teaches skills that help you cope with sudden, intense surges of emotion so you're able to reduce problem behaviors.

DBT has its roots in CBT and uses some of the same techniques, including individual and group therapy sessions, behavior analysis, skills training, and practicing new strategies. But instead of CBT's constant focus on change, DBT works to balance *change* and *acceptance*.

Change and acceptance sound like opposites, which is where the name "dialectical" comes from. It means examining contradictory ideas or facts in a way to resolve something that seems like a contradiction.

Everybody experiences dialectical situations, though we don't call them that. We call them "the challenge of balancing home and work" or "the struggle of meeting the needs of those we love without abandoning our own needs" and "tempering passionate feelings with logical thought."

DBT uses strategies that reflect acceptance and validation of your abilities right now, and combines that acceptance with behavior therapy techniques that help you improve your abilities.

Let's say your daughter is so anxious about going to school that she refuses to get out of bed. No matter what you try, every morning ends in tears, tantrums, or both. She's missed most days of school this semester.

In DBT, the therapist helps your daughter analyze her thoughts and behaviors and figure out alternative ones. At the same time, the DBT therapist openly accepts your daughter's anxiety and acknowledges that refusing to get out of bed is a strategy that works—while continuing to present other strategies that can work, too.

This shifting back and forth between change-accept-change validates your daughter's experience—she *is* severely anxious, and she has by instinct figured out a way to alleviate that anxiety—without losing sight of the need for her to develop better ways to cope with her school anxiety.

When your daughter's DBT therapist validates her anxiety and behavior, it does not mean the therapist approves of the behavior. The therapist can acknowledge that your daughter's behavior makes sense considering her situation and point of view but doesn't have to agree that skipping school is the best solution.

In the course of her DBT, your daughter learns and practices self-validation and self-acceptance skills as well as new behavioral strategies. The goal of this combined approach is to develop self-awareness and skills that she can apply in any area of her life. Once she's learned better ways to deal with her school anxiety, she'll be able to apply the same process to finding and using better strategies to handle her anxiety in other situations (going to Girl Scout meetings or falling asleep by herself, for example).

## PSYCHODYNAMIC THERAPY

Psychodynamic therapy helps the person gain insight into unconscious, internal conflicts that may be causing dysfunctional or unwanted behaviors. The limited research on psychodynamic therapy's effectiveness suggests that it isn't particularly effective in treating depression nor is it suitable for treating bipolar disorder. It may be useful for parents or other family members by helping to raise awareness of family history, dynamics, or other issues that may be contributing to the already difficult task of raising a child or teen who has bipolar disorder.

The basic premise of psychodynamic therapy is that everyone has an unconscious or subconscious mind that holds on to feelings that are difficult to face. Instead of confronting these feelings, we find ways to keep them hidden from ourselves. The defense mechanisms help suppress the painful feelings but can cause problems themselves. The goal of psychodynamic therapy is to allow the client to access the feelings in a safe environment, experience the true feelings, and resolve the inner conflict, which in turn improves overall functioning.

## INTERPERSONAL THERAPY AND IPSRT

Interpersonal therapy (IPT), as its name implies, focuses on the relationships your child has with those who are important in his life: you, his siblings, other family members, peers, and friends. IPT explores the connections between these significant relationships and the bipolar symptoms. Its underlying premise is that the symptoms occur within a social and interpersonal context, and for symptoms to improve, we have to understand that context.

IPT grew out of psychodynamic therapy but unlike the psychodynamic approach, IPT emphasizes how the current relationships and social environment cause, aggravate, or maintain symptoms. Because it focuses on the here-and-now and usually addresses only one or two problem areas at a time, it's a short-term therapy. In the early sessions, you, your child, or both and the therapist decide which areas would be most helpful in alleviating symptoms. During the rest of the sessions, you'll work toward resolving those agreed-upon areas.

IPT has an element of psychoeducational therapy, too, since part of the therapist's job is to help your child learn about the nature of his illness and how his symptoms are expressed in his life and relationships.

IPT was originally developed to treat depression in adults and is now used in both original and modified forms to treat bipolar and other disorders. A recent modification developed by Ellen Frank adds social rhythm therapy (SRT) to IPT to create IPSRT (interpersonal and social rhythm therapy).

The SRT component addresses the importance of "life hygiene" in managing bipolar disorder. We know that kids with bipolar (and adults, too) do much better if they establish and maintain good routines for sleeping, eating, and the other "social rhythms" of everyday life. Disruptions in these rhythms can precipitate or worsen bipolar symptoms, such as when sleep deprivation triggers mania.

SRT incorporates behavioral and psychoeducational approaches and in many ways is similar to the early stages of CBT. Early in IPSRT, treatment focuses on behavioral interventions and scheduling activities to establish and regulate social rhythms—the SRT elements. As your child becomes better at following the daily routine, the focus shifts more to the IP side, working on the connections between interpersonal relationships and bipolar symptoms. Throughout, the therapist helps your child understand how changes in daily routines and the quality of significant relationships can affect his mood.

## FAMILY THERAPY AND FAMILY-FOCUSED THERAPY

Family therapy and family-focused therapy involve all members of the nuclear or extended family, including the patient. The therapist works with family members to improve relationships, educate them about the disorder, and train them in communication and problem-solving skills.

When someone in a family has a chronic illness, the family as a whole develops ways to deal with the illness. Your "family system," whether it's just you and your kid or an extended, multigenerational clan, learns, changes, and grows as if it were a unique being responding to everyone within it and the world around it. Some responses—parents figuring out better ways to communicate with each other, for example—are positive, strengthen the family, and support the person who's ill. Others—blaming a family member for all the problems, for example—aren't helpful and create more problems than they solve.

In family therapy and family-focused therapy, the goal isn't to pluck someone from the system, fix them, and plunk them back into place; the goal is to find ways to improve how the system as a whole works. Family system problems typically involve a combination of habits, old wounds, and unawareness. Family therapists pay particular attention to what's happening between family members, as opposed to what's happening with one specific person. The therapist helps family members recognize and understand how they react and respond to each other, guides them to better alternatives, and supports them as they make changes.

Suppose your family has been coping with your son's rage storms and other bipolar symptoms for a long time, but finally, you've found a meds combination that stabilizes his mood.

Despite that, there's still a lot of discord in the family. His sister baits and berates him until he blows up. Dad is on his case for losing his temper but ignores the sibling taunting that triggers it. Mom wonders if the meds are helping at all; things sure don't seem any different.

In this simple example, the sister may have so much pent-up anger from putting up with her brother for so long that she can't resist sarcasm and put-downs. Dad's so used to his son exploding for no reason that it doesn't occur to him that there might be a reason now. Mom is so busy trying to keep the peace that she doesn't notice that her son's symptoms have improved.

The therapist will help the family members untangle their roles, reactions, and interactions and overcome the negative patterns they've developed, replacing them with better ones.

Family-focused therapy targets high levels of emotion, especially criticism and hostility, and tends to incorporate more psychoeducational therapy, but both approaches strive to create a better functioning home environment by improving communication, solving family problems, and increasing understanding about and building skills to deal with special family situations, including mental illness.

## A NOTE ABOUT RELAPSES

*Keri attends a therapeutic boarding school. Her mood had been stable for many months and, thanks to the intensive counseling and support possible in a specialized residential program, she'd made great progress. She wanted to decrease one of her meds to see if it would help ease a side effect. Under close supervision, she lowered her daily Seroquel dose by only 25 milligrams. It was enough to destabilize her mood. She discovered that despite strong support from her treatment team, she*

*couldn't use the skills she'd worked so hard to learn; her bipolar symp-*
*toms outweighed everything else. She returned to her original Seroquel*
*dose, and as her mood stabilized, she was once again able to use those*
*skills.*

Many illnesses are treated with a combination of medication and therapy. For some of them (anxiety and depression are two of the most common), with lots of therapy and support, you might be able to gradually discontinue meds and stay healthy. In others (and bipolar is certainly in this group), your child will probably need meds even if she's learned better skills and has superb insight about herself.

Bipolar symptoms can break through although her mood has been stable on a particular mix of meds for a while. Symptoms can flare up when you're adjusting meds, trying for a better result. Without meds, she will most likely have a complete relapse, and all the symptoms will come back, even if psychotherapy has helped her.

If you have asthma, your body never learns "how not to wheeze" and unfortunately, that's largely true for bipolar, too. Whether it appears in adults or children, bipolar most often seems to be a chronic medical condition, although the course can vary considerably from person to person. Therapy and all the work you do as a family can help your child learn important skills and improve behavior, but *knowing* how to use the skills and *being able* to use them are two separate things. As a parent or other caregiver, be prepared for the long haul: ups and downs, medication and therapy, good and bad.

# Chapter 9

# INVISIBLE ELEPHANTS

## EDUCATION, ADVOCACY, AND IEPS

*When I feel bad, frustrated, at school especially, I try to keep working, push through it. I'd say to other kids, it's not scary, and meds and therapy are good things.*

ALEX, AGE SEVEN, DIAGNOSED AGE SIX

You've probably heard the phrase "the elephant in the living room." It's the big thing that everybody knows is there but nobody wants to talk about. Everybody avoids it as best they can, stepping around it, dodging the elephant patties, trying not to get stepped on. But no matter how hard you pretend it isn't there, it still takes up a lot of space and affects everything and everyone. Pretty soon, everyone is behaving in ways that don't make sense—and won't make sense until they admit that there really is a ten-ton pachyderm in their midst.

You're already well aware of one potential elephant: bipolar and bipolar plus. Mental health is a common living room elephant. People don't understand it and don't want to deal with it. They may not believe that mental illness or brain disorders exist, especially in children. They can't see the elephant—your child looks "normal," so they expect her to act "normal"—and any struggles your child has are blamed on easier suspects: parents, home life, willful misbehavior. You can see the elephant, but it's invisible to many others.

The other invisible elephant isn't in your living room; it's in the school system. In many respects, our school systems are incredible and wonderful; most people don't think there's an elephant anywhere in sight. Most people have never experienced the challenges you and your child face every day.

"No Child Left Behind" sounds great, but all too often, children with bipolar are left behind, their education thwarted by the very institutions that are supposed to be providing it.

In the United States, every child is entitled to a free appropriate public education, and that includes the kids who look "normal" but aren't: those who have invisible disabilities such as bipolar, ADHD, anxiety disorders, and learning disabilities.

There are good teachers out there, good schools and administrators, too, but when it comes to providing the services these kids need, they are often the exception, not the rule. There are reasons (and lots of excuses) why it is hard for students to get the services they need. Money is tight, classrooms are crowded. Teachers aren't trained in these types of disabilities. Problem behaviors are blamed on bad parenting or a bad kid instead of recognized as symptoms of a serious illness. Lack of behavior problems at school is seen as proof that parents are overreacting or trying to get something their child doesn't need or deserve. These and other roadblocks can make obtaining a free appropriate public education for your child difficult—but not impossible.

You must be an active advocate for your child. You might also need to bring in an outside advocate to help you find and obtain appropriate educational solutions.

Effective advocates, whether parent, volunteer, or professional, know and understand the federal laws that apply to special education. They have ideas about the educational approaches and settings that may work best for your child, and they're open to suggestions proposed by teachers and other professionals. They are familiar with state and federal agencies that might provide programs, funding, or other relevant services. They know that the focus must always be on what best meets the needs of *this child.*

Children and teens who have bipolar are often eligible for—and need—accommodations, modifications, programs, and support services that are accessed through the state's and school district's special education departments. Educating kids who have special needs is a large and complex topic, but the basics are the same for every child, regardless of the type of disability. This chapter covers the basic process: what to expect, where to begin, what to do when you hit a roadblock. For more information, see Appendix E.

## THIS BRAIN IS STILL GROWING

The brains of children and teens are still developing, and each child develops at his or her own rate. That's why one child is ready to read earlier than another. In addition to individual variations in development, children with bipolar are more likely to be on multiple medications, which can affect their cognitive, or thinking, ability. Recent studies show that school-age children with bipolar did worse on tests of attention, verbal memory, working memory, and executive function compared to healthy children, *even when their mood symptoms were stable.* Kids who had both bipolar and ADHD performed even more poorly on attention and executive function tests. In other words, the cognitive and learning problems were present whether or not a child was on medication; meds did not fix these problems even when they did stabilize the child's mood. These studies reinforce the importance of—and need for—educational interventions and supports to address specific cognitive and learning challenges.

The educational needs of children with bipolar disorder are many, varied, and complex. A common misunderstanding in schools is that bipolar is only about moods and emotional disturbance. Teachers may not be aware that your child's disorganization, forgetfulness, distractibility, and social skills problems are part of bipolar, too. To design an educational program that best meets your child's needs, the evaluation must include thorough, detailed assessments for executive function, visual and auditory processing, memory, and social skills.

## WHAT TO EXPECT

Figuring out why your child is having trouble at school and what to do about it seems like it should be a simple and straightforward process. A few tests, fill out some paperwork, and you're on your way.

But, like most things concerning kids with bipolar disorder, the reality is often much more complex.

Evaluations and test results contradict each other. There are disagreements—between you and the school, between teachers, between specialists—about diagnoses, appropriate support services, and necessary accommodations. You want what's best for your child; the school, juggling the needs of many children, worries about its budget. Just when things seem to be going well, symptoms reemerge or meds change or something else knocks everything out of whack.

Expect frustration, exhaustion, and emotional upheaval; they're common and absolutely appropriate.

You may feel as if you're alone in your struggle to find educational solutions for your child, but rest assured, you are not alone, and neither is your child. You may feel as if it's you against the world (or at least against the school system), but you don't have to face all those "official experts" by yourself.

Be warned that this will never be easy. There will be good days, days when everything works and your child is happy and learning and obviously benefiting from his educational setting. There will also be horrible days, days when the school blames you, days when the teacher tells you he's a bad kid, or not sick, or any number of other things you know aren't true. Days when your child is miserable or too sick to stay in school. Days when you break down in the car and cry all the way home, and days when you break down and cry in a school meeting (which is sometimes worse, but not always).

There is tension and conflict and worry.

All of this is normal. Sometimes it's even productive: Out of the tension and conflict, creative, effective solutions are born.

The way through the challenges is to stay focused on this fundamental question:

*What best meets the needs of my child?*

Sometimes you'll rephrase the question to address a particular situation. For example, if the principal says your daughter ought to be expelled from school or pulled out of her beloved science class because she had a meltdown in language arts, you ask, calmly and professionally (you may be gritting your teeth or ready to tear your hair out, but you *can* do this), "*How* does this best meet the needs of my child?"

Everything must come back to this fundamental question. It really is the goal. The goal isn't a therapeutic boarding school a thousand miles away—unless that's what best meets her needs. The goal isn't avoiding special ed or support services—unless that best meets her needs.

The goal is to identify the things that are getting in the way of your child's education—her *needs,* which are different from those of kids who don't have these emotional and cognitive challenges—and to figure out *what* will help her learn and grow despite those needs.

## WHERE TO BEGIN

You've already taken the first step, though you may not realize it. The first step is asking why your child is struggling so much at school.

Like any parent, you know your child is smart and creative, that he loves some topics and struggles with others. You probably have a good sense of his learning style. The teacher says he ought to be able to do all the things the other kids in his class do, from being polite and respectful to reading at grade level and keeping his work organized.

But he isn't able to, and you've identified (or are in the process of identifying) one important reason. The medical diagnosis of bipolar disorder (and any plus disorders), while scary, explains a lot. It isn't the entire answer, but it's a piece of the answer.

The next step depends on whether the school has noticed anything's amiss. You and the teacher may have already talked about problems and concerns, either casually or in formal parent-teacher conferences. Such conversations are important and useful, but they are not enough to begin special ed services for your child. For that, your child must have a full, comprehensive, individual evaluation.

*Written* requests and consent forms are the next step. You, the state education agency or other state agency, or the school district (through your child's school or special ed department) can request an evaluation for your child.

If you've received a written notice from the school requesting permission to evaluate your child for specific disabilities, your next step is to sign and date the notice and return it.

If you haven't received a written notice from the school, your next step is to request, in writing, an evaluation for your child. Sign and date your request and keep a copy of it for your records. The school should respond with a consent form for you to sign, date, and return.

> Include the date on *all* notices and forms—the school must take action within time frames specified by state and federal guidelines.

The consent form should include a list of the tests and evaluations the school wants to administer. If you don't understand what some or all of them are, what they're for, or how they'll be administered, ask! Make an appointment with the specialists who will be giving the test to your child and ask them to explain what they'll be doing and what they hope to learn from the results.

If there's a particular test or type of evaluation you want included, list it on your "request for evaluation" letter, and if you discover an evaluation that you should have included but didn't, add it to the consent form along with a signed and dated letter noting the request.

In addition to the school's evaluations, you can ask for an independent evaluation. This may be necessary if you don't agree with the results of the school's assessment or if you believe the school's assessments aren't sufficient to show a clear picture of the challenges your child faces.

The assessments your school provides may be inadequate for a number of reasons, including conflict of interest (the school must address any problems the assessments reveal, which can be an incentive to administer fewer or less comprehensive tests); lack of qualified personnel (for example, neuropsychological assessment is an important test schools should but often don't do because they don't have anyone on staff qualified to administer it); and lack of knowledge (the school may not be aware of the importance of assessing executive function, for example).

If you're not sure what tests to ask for or what the school's suggested tests will tell you, speak with your child's psychologist, psychiatrist, or an educational advocate. You can also find more information in the books and Web sites listed in the "More Information and Resources for School Support Services, Special Education, and IEPs" section in Appendix E.

The school can do many different kinds of evaluations. These are paid for by the school, not by you. Additional testing or independent evaluations may be covered by the school, by the parents, or shared between the two. If there's a medical reason for the test, for example, if the test results might lead to starting or changing medication, your health insurance might cover the cost. Even if you have to pay for an evaluation out of your own pocket, it can be worth it, especially if the school's results don't mesh with what you know about your child. The cost of medical exams, for example, the doctor's evaluation that led to your child's diagnosis of bipolar, are your responsibility and are not covered by the school.

*Midway through fall semester, Mica's fifth-grade teacher confirmed his mom's worries. She'd been teaching for a long time and had seen almost every problem a kid could have, and Mica was definitely atypical. She recommended that Mica have a thorough neuropsychological evaluation to assess his executive skills, working and short-term memory, and auditory and visual processing abilities. Three months and nine-plus hours of evaluations later, Mica's mom, Bethany, had a complete write-up of the results and a challenging set of diagnoses. The top two problems were pediatric bipolar disorder and Asperger's syndrome.*

*Bethany thought she'd feel relieved once she had a diagnosis— she'd been trying to understand what was going on with Mica since he was very young—but instead of relieved, she felt completely overwhelmed. Her first impulse was to not let anyone know about her son's diagnosis, especially at school. She was embarrassed and worried about Mica being "labeled." She met with Mica's teacher, who reassured her and explained that the diagnosis was actually protective. The diagnosis was the door to support services, and the recommendations, tied to Mica's evaluation results, told them where to begin.*

You'll need to include written documentation from your doctor regarding your child's diagnosis. Schools, including general and special ed teachers, administrators, social workers, speech and language therapists, and school psychologists, are not qualified or authorized to make medical diagnoses or prescribe medications. This means that although certain school professionals can identify and diagnose learning disabilities, they cannot diagnose your child with bipolar disorder, anxiety disorders, ADHD, conduct disorder, oppositional defiant disorder, or autism spectrum disorder, nor can they tell you what medications your child should take. But often, they do need to know and understand the medical diagnosis in order to understand your child's educational needs. Even though you may feel reluctant to divulge your child's medical information, in many cases, it is important to do so.

Talk with your clinician about the wisdom of being frank with the school. Usually, disclosing your child's diagnosis opens the door to needed services, but not always. In some schools, the bipolar diagnosis, especially if your child has mood symptoms at school, might block entry to LD programs. This situation arises when school personnel don't know much about bipolar and may be aggravated by stigma associated with mental illness or outright prejudice. If this is true for your child's school, you may be better off disclosing only the information concerning your child's learning disabilities.

The school is required by law to keep the information in your child's records confidential, which means they may not release any of the information or discuss it with anyone unless you have given them written permission to do so.

The information you, the school, and other specialists gather during this initial assessment helps determine whether your child is eligible for special education services. It also identifies how your child learns: her learning style, interests, and strengths, as well as her unique needs.

## KEEP RECORDS!

Document everything, and set up a file system.

Documentation serves several purposes. First, it is a record of what you've requested and when, so that you can verify (or challenge) the school's actions. Second, it will help you monitor your child's progress and help identify problem areas or issues that your child is encountering as well as highlight things that are working well. Third, it helps ensure that your child's IEP (individualized educational program) is being implemented properly. Fourth, it helps you prepare for meetings: IEP meetings, manifestation and due process hearings, mediation, and anything else that surfaces during your child's schooling.

Your system doesn't have to be fancy. Parents have used everything from the "big box" approach (the current year's information is in an easily accessible file folder, and past years are in a big box, with older stuff on the bottom, newer materials on the top) to three-ring binders (one or more per year) to electronic scans of paper documents stored on computers. You can even hire someone to keep your records organized and accurate for you. Use whatever works for you.

Save everything, and put everything in writing. If you talk to the school on the phone, make a note of the date and time of the call, the reason for the call, and the name of the person you spoke with. If you visit with the teacher or specialist informally (chatting about how things went that day at school, for example) or in a formal meeting, take notes, either during or immediately after. Include the date and time, who was there, what you talked about, what action is supposed to happen next, who's going to do it, how you'll know if it's done, and what the next step after that will be. Include enough detail so that the note will make sense if you read it a month later. (You think you'll remember everything, but you won't. Write it down, put it in the file.) Not sure you can take notes at a formal meeting? Either record the meeting or bring someone along to take notes for you.

In addition to the forms, notices, correspondence, and meeting notes, your files should include a copy of your child's entire school record (anything the school has that has your child's name on it); samples of schoolwork (homework and class work); copies of assessments and evaluations (including the results and explanations of results); report cards; progress reports; any other reports issued by the school, including disciplinary reports; and, once it's created, your child's IEP.

## CREATING YOUR CHILD'S EDUCATIONAL PLAN

Evaluations can take up to six weeks, not counting school vacations. Once they're completed, it's time for your first big meeting: the initial IEP team meeting.*

*IEP* stands for *individualized educational program.* It's the document that explains why your child needs services, what those services are, how you'll know if the services are helping your child, and the plan for providing the services. You, your child when appropriate, and the other members of the IEP team create the IEP for your child.

Before the first meeting, the school creates a report describing the results of the evaluations. You should receive this report at least forty-eight hours before the meeting. This is true for other meetings, too—anytime there are new test results to review, you should have the information about the tests and results at least forty-eight hours before meeting with the school to discuss the results. This gives you a chance to review the report and its recommendations before the meeting.

The report should include results from independent or

---

*Some school districts call these *IEPT meetings* (the "T" is for *team*).

outside evaluations, too, provided that you gave permission for those results to be sent to the school. If the outside evaluation results aren't included in the report, or if you notice anything else that's incorrect or missing, contact the school right away so that they can get the missing information to other team members, too.

The IEP meeting will include everyone who is involved with your child's education: at least one of your child's regular education teachers; at least one of his special ed teachers or other qualified person who provides special education services to him; a representative of the school district who is qualified to provide or supervise providing special ed services and who knows about the curriculum and the district's resources; someone who can explain what the evaluation results mean in terms of your child's education; the student, when appropriate; and other specialists as needed. For example, if you need a translator, the district must provide one; if the evaluations show that your daughter has dyslexia, the reading specialist should attend the IEP meeting.

If your child is in middle, junior high, or senior high school, she probably has different regular education teachers for different classes. It's beneficial—to the teachers, who learn about the student and why the items in the IEP are needed, and to the team, which benefits from the additional observations and input—to have as many of the other teachers attend as possible, but their attendance isn't required by law. Also, "attending" doesn't necessarily mean "showing up in person and sitting in the room." People can "attend" via phone and videoconferencing.

The IEP meeting also—and most importantly—includes you, the parents. At least one parent should attend the meeting. It's great if the other parent or stepparents actively involved in the care of your child can attend the meeting, too.

You can also bring anyone else to the meeting you want to bring: an advocate, the psychiatrist, a friend for emotional support, a note-taker. If you bring the psychiatrist or therapist, or if your advocate is fee-based, you will have to pay their fee. In special circumstances, if the school requests that your psychiatrist or other mental health clinician attend, the school may be willing to pay the fees (it never hurts to ask). You do not pay for the school's personnel or specialists.

The purpose of the IEP meeting is to figure out what best meets the educational needs of your child. From this meeting (and subsequent meetings, if you don't get everything done during the first meeting), you'll confirm whether or not your child is eligible for special education services and develop a plan addressing her unique educational strengths and weaknesses.

During the IEP meeting, you and the other members of your child's IEP team will go through the information you've all gathered: the evaluation and test results; observations and records from you and the teachers about behavior, learning style, special interests, strengths, weaknesses or problem areas, things that trigger meltdowns, situations where symptoms seem to ease up or worsen; and medical information, including diagnosis and medications. Information about your child's current school performance—progress reports, report cards, and so on—also goes into the mix. Your child's input should be included, too. During initial meetings and when your child is young, you'll provide this information, and as your child matures and begins to learn to advocate for herself, she can attend the IEP meetings and contribute directly.

*Educational needs* are more than the classic three Rs. Social skills, emotional development, and behavior management are major components of education. They are just as important as the intellectual and academic aspects and should be addressed in the IEP.

Educational needs are more than what happens during the six or so hours your child is in school, too. Homework wars, meltdowns every day after school, and severe difficulty rousing in the morning all happen outside the formal school day, and all are part of the whole environment that has an impact on your child's ability to learn—and must, therefore, be covered in the IEP.

All of the assessment information, including medical diagnosis and any independent evaluation results, should be recorded in the IEP.

During the rest of the meeting, you and the other team members will discuss goals and objectives and how those will be reached. This information becomes part of the IEP, too, and includes teaching strategies, curriculum modifications, alternative programs, support services, how and when progress will be monitored, and any other accommodations the IEP team specifies. There are all kinds of accommodations, support services, and alternative approaches that parents and teachers have come up with to provide a free appropriate public education for kids who have bipolar. (See "Yes, You Can!" page 232.) As with regular education, programs, methods, and curriculum should be supported by research.

A common challenge for parents with kids like yours is teachers or other school personnel who are unconvinced that a child needs any accommodations or special ed services because he doesn't cause problems at school and his grades are okay. It is your job, with the help of an advocate or the clinician, if necessary, to enlighten the school professionals.

You know, because he's your kid and you know him better than anyone else does, that he holds it together at school because he's so afraid of losing it in front of the other kids. It's a tremendous strain on him. Sometimes he's so focused on holding it together that he misses half of what the teacher says. The only reason his grades are as good as they are is because he's so smart or because he's working extra hard. In fact, his grades ought to be a lot better—and would be, if he didn't struggle with his illness every day.

You also know the cost of his schooltime efforts: He has major meltdowns every day after school. Doing homework is a nightmare. What control he's been able to muster during the day is gone, his energy depleted.

This is a good example of how something that seems to be outside of school is actually part of the bigger educational picture. Frequent after-school meltdowns and homework wars or, conversely, extreme anxiety or major battles before school are in part a response to the during-school environment.

Once you've established that these "outside" behaviors are part of the educational needs that must be addressed in the IEP, you and the IEP team can develop accommodations and strategies that consider the entire educational environment, not just the part of it that exists inside the school building.

Homework is one of the biggest problems, and we often recommend cutting down or eliminating it entirely, without penalty. In other words, your child won't lose points or grades because she didn't do her homework.

This suggestion rattles some teachers (and some parents). They don't like it—after all, homework is important!

Well, maybe yes, maybe no. For a variety of reasons, homework loads, even in the early elementary school years, are much heavier than they used to be. A lot of homework is simply repetition that doesn't further learning. It's make-work more than expand-your-knowledge work. If your child needs practice in a particular subject, there are methods other than homework to build proficiency.

For some children, including some who have bipolar, homework isn't a big deal. For others, homework is not appropriate, or not appropriate in the quantity and form typically used in today's classrooms. One tip-off that homework is counterproductive is if your child scores As and Bs on quizzes and exams but has Ds in the class because of missing homework assignments. Another clue is if he's having frequent severe rage storms after school. Decreased or no homework is a valid accommodation for these children. You can set up accommodations for homework and other tasks so they're flexible: When your child's illness stabilizes, she may be able to do more or all of her homework, and if symptoms flare, she does less or no homework.

Since what goes on during school can have a strong impact on what happens outside of school and what happens outside of school can affect what happens during school, you and the IEP team need to keep open eyes and open minds about the school environment. What would make it easier, less stressful, more positive, and safer at school for your child? Not "easier" as in watering down the curriculum—that's a different issue—but what would make it easier for your child to be at school and have a fair chance to learn? Would it help if he could start later in the day? For kids who are groggy from meds or have the night owl sleep pattern so common in bipolar, beginning school at ten instead of eighty-thirty might enable them to function better through the rest of the day. Would it help if she could go home earlier? Maybe a half day of school is what's best for now, or a combination of in-school classes and a homebound tutor. Perhaps a completely different setting in a specialized classroom in a public school or a charter school that has more flexibility and creativity would be a better fit.

There's a lot to consider during an IEP meeting. Most of the time, meetings (any kind) are set up to last a certain length of time. One school of thought says that IEP meetings, whether the first or subsequent ones, should be open-ended, and nobody goes home until you've gone through the entire thing. That may work, especially in cases where you're dealing with a few well-known specific issues. For things as complex as bipolar and bipolar plus, it can take a long time to cover all the material and hash out a plan. No matter how important the meeting is, it's hard to sit through more than a couple of hours. If you're meeting before school, teachers will have to leave for their classes when school begins, and if you're meeting after school, everyone wants to go home for supper.

You might be tempted or pressured by other team members to wrap things up quickly, sign whatever paper they put in front of you, and be done with it.

Don't.

The only thing you should sign during an IEP meeting is the form that lists who attended.

If you don't get everything done today, schedule another meeting to continue the discussion. The next meeting could be after lunch or in a day or two—soon enough that everyone still remembers what you were talking about and you don't have to chew up precious minutes in extensive review. You also want to push for the next meeting as soon as possible because the longer you wait, the longer your child has to wait for the services and programs she needs.

Depending on your school, the IEP may be written up by hand as the meeting progresses, a school staff member will type it, and you'll review it before or during a second meeting. Some schools have the forms in the computer and will enter information during the meeting and print out a "finished IEP" at the end of the meeting. In both cases, what the school gives you often looks like a "done deal": Here's your kid's problems, here's what we're going to do, sign here.

Even though the form looks finished, don't sign it yet. Take it home and read it all the way through. Make sure you understand it, all of it. Do you agree with the goals that have been established? Are the goals and concerns that are important to you included? Is the medical information included and accurate? Do the programs, methods, support services, and accommodations make sense to you? For example, suppose the IEP lists "reading specialist twenty minutes daily" because your son's reading scores are low. You suspect his scores are low because he's so anxious about school he can't concentrate, and it's worse because reading is first thing in the morning when he's extra groggy. The school's recommendation for a reading specialist is not enough. The IEP must address the anxiety and sleep issues, too. Maybe he needs a later start for his school day and a safe place to go if he begins to feel overwhelmed or anxious, as well as a reading specialist.

Once you've carefully reviewed the IEP and are satisfied that it includes the things you and the team agreed to during your discussions, you can sign and date it. The school may have provided two copies, one for you to keep; put the date on that one, too. If not, be sure to get a copy of your signed and dated form from the school to include in your files for future reference.

---

### BRING SNACKS!

One tip that we always recommend for an IEP meeting is to bring food! Teachers often attend these meetings before school or during lunch or their planning period, and they don't have time to eat. By bringing food, you are acknowledging that you understand they are taking extra time out of their day. It encourages a team approach, helps everyone feel valued, and will pay off in the long run for your child.

*Susan Resko, Executive Director,*
*Child & Adolescent Bipolar Foundation*

---

The IEP shouldn't sit on the shelf gathering dust. Copies of it—all of it, not just the goals and objectives page—must be distributed to all your child's teachers, even the gym teacher, and all of your child's teachers are required by law to follow the accommodations, programs, and other directives of the IEP. For example, if your child's IEP specifies no homework, that means no homework—not in math, science, language arts, or any other class. If his IEP says he is to use a calculator for arithmetic, that means he must be allowed to use the calculator for in-class work, homework, and exams.

Your work as your child's advocate isn't done when the IEP is done. Although your child's teachers and other school personnel are required by law to implement the IEP, sometimes they don't receive a copy of it, or they overlook it. They may misunderstand what is required or even refuse to follow it. So, once you have the IEP in place, check in with your child's teachers and counselors to make sure they've received and reviewed it, and that they understand the services and accommodations. Follow up with them occasionally, more often if things aren't improving, and check in with new teachers before school begins each term.

The IEP must be reviewed and updated every year, and every three years, the school must reevaluate your child to determine whether or not she's still eligible for special education services. This *triennial review* is similar in scope to the initial assessment and IEP development. During the annual reviews and the triennial, you'll meet with the IEP team to set new goals and objectives and decide how to build on the progress your child has made. In addition, when your child is ready to make the next big step—elementary school to middle or junior high, from there to high school, and high school to graduation and beyond—you'll also create a transition plan that becomes part of the IEP.

You don't have to wait for a year to review or change the IEP. You can request a review or update whenever you feel it's necessary. You don't have to include all the IEP team members for these interim meetings, only those who are directly involved in the program or accommodation you want to examine or change.

## FAIR DOESN'T MEAN EQUAL

Are you feeling guilty about asking for "special stuff" that probably costs a lot, thinking that by doing so, you're taking away precious resources that others need? Are you hesitant to ask for programs or services that might help your child because you've heard that your school district doesn't have a lot of money? Have you felt the sting of teachers, administrators, or other parents who aren't familiar with IDEA (the special education law), who claim that the school doesn't have to provide a service, or that if they do, they'll have to cut services for other kids, or that it isn't fair that your kid is getting something better, more, or different than other kids get?

*Fair* doesn't mean *equal*. Fair means addressing needs. Fair is exactly what you're trying to do by meeting your child's needs. Most kids don't need extra services. Some need a few, and some need lots. Here's another way to think about "fair": It isn't fair that your child has challenges to deal with that other kids don't have.

You're not looking for equal; you're looking for fair, and a free appropriate public education is *fair.*

Your first responsibility is to your child. Your job is not to solve the school district's real or imagined financial woes. Your job is to advocate for your child so that your child can go to school and have a *fair* chance to learn.

If your school district has such severe financial problems that it cannot offer appropriate services to its students and you want to help remedy that, put your energy into campaigning for better funding, writing grant proposals, getting local businesses to donate supplies and equipment, or anything else you think will help—but do these things after, not before or instead of, advocating for your child.


## ADVICE FOR FINDING AN ADVOCATE

Tami Joia, professional advocate and founder of I.D.E.A.S., a nonprofit advocacy assistance and training organization in Brockton, Massachusetts, says hiring an advocate is just like hiring a plumber: The advocate is working for you, advocating for your child, and you need to ask questions to find out if the advocate is qualified. An advocate who's great for kids with physical disabilities may or may not be a good match for kids who have bipolar or other brain disorders.

Ask a prospective advocate: How long have you been an

advocate? Do you have a specialty? How much experience do you have with kids like mine? What do you know about my child's disabilities (bipolar, bipolar plus, learning disabilities, others), specifically?

If the advocate doesn't know the answers to some of your questions, she should at least know where to go to get the information. You and the advocate need to match the needs caused by your child's disabilities with appropriate services to meet those needs. The advocate must know how to apply IDEA 2004 (Individuals with Disabilities Education Act, reauthorized by the United States Congress in 2004) to your child's specific situation.

When you decide to use an advocate, the advocate should begin by reviewing your child's records—the school records, any evaluation or test results, teachers' assessments, independent evaluations, and medical information. Ideally, you'll have an advocate who's up-to-date on the latest research and other info about bipolar and any other challenges your child has. Experienced advocates also know about the options that are available in your area and farther afield, how different programs are funded, and what those programs offer.

## YES, YOU CAN!

Parents, teachers, advocates, and others have figured out many creative approaches to help kids with bipolar learn and grow. Here's a small sampling.

Reduce or eliminate homework.
Make accommodations for homework or other tasks adjustable so they can flex with and respond to symptoms, medication, etc.
Start school later, leave earlier.
Create and follow a consistent, predictable schedule with plenty of breaks.

Allow extra time to get from one class to the next.

Identify and allow the student to use an "escape valve" spot.

Supplement part-time school attendance (or replace in-class attendance) with homebound (also called home-based) tutoring paid for by the school district.

Create and follow plans for what to do during unstructured time.

Schedule the day so the student can tackle the hardest stuff when they're best able to perform (think about meds, hunger, fatigue, circadian rhythms, and anything else that may help or hinder).

Schedule high-interest classes first thing in the morning.

Allow untimed testing or extra time for taking tests.

Provide a one-on-one aide (paraprofessional) in the classroom.

Provide general life skills instruction.

Provide instruction in finding and using organizational aids (daily planners, timers, etc.).

Provide a playground aide.

Allow ready access to guidance counselor or therapist.

Placement in special class for behavior, learning, or both.

Participate in a social skills group.

Allow relaxed deadlines on long-term projects.

Allow untimed testing in quiet, low-stimulation or low-distraction surroundings.

Use a keyboard instead of writing with pen or pencil.

Create a crisis management plan that includes actions other than calling parent to come collect the student.

Participate in extended school year (ESY).

Participate in summer camp programs that include
educational services.
Placement in specialized schools, including public
charter schools, therapeutic day and residential
schools, and residential treatment centers.

*Christopher's illness is both complex and severe: bipolar with extreme
and rapid mood swings, plus ADHD, anxiety disorders, Asperger's
syndrome, and multiple learning disabilities. He's highly distractible
but stimulant meds make his bipolar symptoms worse. He's been on
many different medications for his bipolar and has frequent symptom
breakthroughs. He has problems with executive functioning (organizing, decision-making, focusing attention), cognitive processing, and
social skills.*

*Samantha, Christopher's mom, says at first, like many parents, she
just wanted her son to fit in, so she hired her first tutor for Christopher
when he was four years old. During the next few years, she realized
that neither the after-school tutors nor the mainstream classroom were
appropriate placements for Christopher, and the school's resource room
placement was worse.*

*Christopher's bipolar certainly complicated his ability to learn, but
Samantha was confident that a comprehensive educational approach
addressing her son's learning problems plus his mood disorder would
be more effective than either the limited services the school was offering
or a solely therapeutic approach. She challenged the school's decision,
pursuing the case through the courts and ultimately setting a precedent
for others in their state, and put together a creative solution for her
son's education. (See "Christopher's Schedule," below.)*

*The rationale behind the subjects and educational approaches in
Christopher's program comes both from the advice of the instructors
and therapists Samantha has found and her own research about methods that help remediate the kinds of problems Christopher has (executive functioning, for example). As an outgrowth of her commitment to
finding research-based programs for Christopher and professionals
who can provide those programs, Samantha has hosted training sessions and workshops for other educators.*

*She hasn't stopped there. Even though her son will continue his education outside the mainstream classroom, Samantha continues to fight for the educational rights of children who have severe illnesses and disabilities.*

***Christopher's Schedule:*** *Christopher's schooling is a unique "home-based" program, though the only time he's actually at home for classes is when he's in a bipolar crisis. His schooling takes place seven days a week, Monday through Sunday, year-round, except for the one to two days each month when he* and his parents travel to a teaching hospital to meet with several specialists. His mom drives him to each place each day. Christopher's course credits are planned, tracked, and approved through Clonlara School, which is an organization that services homeschooling families throughout the United States (www. clonlara.org).*

*Five days a week (Monday through Friday), Samantha drives Christopher to the public library nearest their home, about five miles away. At the library, in a small study room, Christopher meets with his math teacher for an hour. They have access to all the library resources, including computers, the Internet, and books at every level and on practically every topic.*

*Next up is the Lindamood-Bell Learning Center (www.lblp.com/ learningcenters), whose sensory-cognitive programs have been approved by the U.S. Department of Education for working with expressive disorders. Christopher spends two hours with two different instructors who use a variety of methods to teach math and language arts.*

*On Mondays, they leave Lindamood-Bell and drive for half an hour to Christopher's art class, held at the instructor's house. The art teacher has inside and outside studios, and they work in all media— ceramics, painting, woodworking, and more—for three and a half hours.*

*At the end of the day on Monday and mid-afternoon on Wednesday and Friday, they go from Lindamood-Bell to a different public library and meet for an hour and a half with an instructor Christopher calls his "games teacher." The instructor uses chess, poker, Rummikub, Scrabble, pool, and other games to help Christopher improve his executive and cognitive functioning skills. Samantha suggested this approach after learning about research that showed improved cognitive functioning and higher level thinking skills in adult Alzheimer and brain injury patients who played these types of games. Ninety minutes of American history follows the games sessions on Wednesday and Friday.*

*On Thursdays, they start the math hour at the public library later in the morning, then spend two hours at Lindamood-Bell in the early afternoon, followed by a session with a cognitive-behavioral therapist, and round out the day with an hour of American history at the library.*

*On Saturday, Christopher has another ninety-minute games session mid-morning followed by ninety minutes of American history. On Sunday, he has ninety minutes of language arts.*

*They're about to add two more classes to Christopher's schedule. First up is American Sign Language, which meets the foreign language credit requirement for high school, provides yet another way to work Christopher's visual motor, fine motor, and nonverbal skills, and provides an opportunity for him to meet children who have disabilities different from his own. The ASL class will meet for about an hour on Sunday afternoons.*

*Soon after that, Samantha will add Feuerstein Instrumental Enrichment for an hour each day. This program, developed by Professor Reuven Feuerstein (www.icelp.org, www.iriinc.us), is another research-based method that may help correct some of Christopher's deficient cognitive functions and enhance his capacity to learn more effectively in a variety of situations.*

*In addition to Christopher's classes and therapy appointments, his parents provide a wide variety of enrichment activities whenever possible. They go on weekly and monthly field trips to museums, galleries, and anything else that may increase his ability to learn.*

*Samantha says, "I'm letting Christopher lead us. We've seen tremendous growth—he's continuing to mature in all areas—and we'll keep doing this unless it slows down or plateaus. It's hard when other eighteen-year-olds are graduating from high school and going off to college. He's not there yet, and I won't give up allowing him to learn and grow.*

*"You can't stop fighting for them. I have to plan on the bad, but I*

*won't stop dreaming for a wonderful future for him and working to help him get there."*

*Eva is just as committed as Samantha to finding the best education for her daughter, but as a single mother who works full-time, she can't afford a long legal battle with the school or to spend each day shuttling her daughter to different places. Meeting her daughter's educational needs took strong advocacy and creativity. She contacted the public library and her state's department of education to learn about her legal options, consulted by phone with a nonprofit legal agency, and successfully persuaded the school to pay for a more comprehensive evaluation of her daughter's learning difficulties. For several years, her daughter's educational program has included a combination of mainstream classes with a variety of accommodations, an accelerated math class, daily sessions with a language specialist, permission to go to the school library or the guidance counselor's office whenever she feels too anxious to stay in class, and twice-weekly sessions with a mentor from a nearby university who comes to the school.*

## THERAPEUTIC BOARDING SCHOOLS

*Keri, who was diagnosed with pediatric bipolar disorder when she was twelve years old, has always had problems with mood. Her relatives began to call her the "Queen of Mean" when she was a toddler. Her mom developed adult-onset bipolar a few years after Keri became ill. Keri's now in eleventh grade at a therapeutic boarding school.*

*"I remember being pissed off and not believing that meds or therapy would help you. It was okay to see this therapist because I wanted to please my mom and also get her off my back. I was worried that if I didn't go to therapy, it might put my mom back in the hospital, she'd have a relapse, and maybe we'd both be in the hospital and everything would be worse. I decided it wasn't a big deal to pop a few pills.*

*"It took some time for the meds to work. I still have a hard time believing a certain pill will help you. Every med has a side effect; I thought it would be easier.*

*"I'm not sure what I think about treatment, because so much has*

*happened. It's hard to remember what it was like before meds, but I know I'm doing better than I was two months ago. I think that I'm stable now.*

*"Sometimes, I worry that they'll never let me out of here. I don't want to go too soon, but I don't want to be here forever. We delayed my high school graduation a year, so that takes pressure off; it gives me plenty of time to ease back into whatever's next.*

*"I think about my goals for the future a lot. I want to go to college, I want to study business and fashion design and make lots of money. For my first year, I'll stay around here and then definitely transfer to someplace else.*

*"I'd tell other kids to maybe give meds a try. I don't like saying that, because I never got a chance to be stable on my own. For my whole life, I'll be on meds. I don't want to think about that. But it feels good to be stable and not all over the place."*

*Least Restrictive Environments* (LREs) range from full days in a mainstream classroom to therapeutic boarding schools or residential treatment centers—schools where your child lives full-time while going to school.

Sending your child away to school is a big decision. It isn't the first choice for most families, and for most children, it won't be necessary. Most of those who do attend won't spend all their remaining school years as a resident of the school.

Boarding schools aren't your school district's first choice, either; they're an expensive educational option. Your home district will want to try other, less restrictive environments first, and most will not authorize a residential placement without a fight.

Once you've determined that your child does need a therapeutic boarding school, you need to find a school that's a good match for you and your child. Therapeutic schools vary in many ways, from student ages and types of challenges to philosophies about medication and approach to discipline.

F. L. Chamberlain School in Middleboro, Massachusetts, is

a therapeutic school for eleven- to twenty-two-year-olds. It is both a day school (students live at home and commute) and a residential, or boarding, school (students live in small, cottage-style dormitories on campus).

Larry Mutty, admissions director, emphasizes that Chamberlain is a school, not just a therapy program. Students here take the same core subjects that children and teens study in mainstream schools. They can also take topics outside of the core subjects—ocean biology or equestrian study, for example. Chamberlain is a fully accredited high school, which means its students can earn their high school diplomas here. The academic calendar is similar to mainstream middle and high schools, too.

About half of Chamberlain's students go on to college, often attending smaller colleges that have built-in supports for students. Some students participate in pre-vocational training such as internships and work co-op programs and enter the workforce when they leave Chamberlain. Others transition from Chamberlain's program back to their home-district school. The ultimate goals for Chamberlain students are independence and autonomy.

So far, this sounds pretty much like a regular school. What's different?

Therapy is part of the fabric of the school. The school understands and takes advantage of each student's individual learning style. Class sizes are small (eight students and two teachers per class) and most classes include more than one grade level.

About 80% of Chamberlain's students have IEPs, and all or part of their school cost is paid for by their home district. The other 20% are private students whose families pay their way. All of the residential and most of the day students attend a thirty-six-day summer session in addition to the regular fall and spring school terms.

Clinicians—master's degree and above—work with individual students and different groups of students and use a variety of therapeutic approaches. On-site psychiatric care is included in the tuition. Ninety percent of the students take meds, and within the safe, closely supervised, and tightly coordinated residential school setting, it's easier to explore the effectiveness of different types and dosages of medications.

Larry Mutty strongly recommends that parents considering a therapeutic residential school investigate several schools. Visit them, ask questions, and look for what you think will work for your child.

Questions to ask include:

- What's the staff turnover? (How long have teachers, residential counselors, overnight staff, and other staff worked for the school, on average?)

- What are the teacher credentials?

- What are the credentials and training for others who will be working with my child?

- What are the discipline policies, including policies regarding expulsion?

- What is the school's focus? (Some schools focus more on emotionally fragile children, others on children who are recovering from abuse or trauma, still others on those who have severe conduct disorder or criminal behavior challenges.)

- What is the school's approach, policy, and philosophy regarding therapeutic approaches? regarding medication?

- How will the school coordinate care with your current doctor, therapist, or other team members?

- How does the school address safety issues?

- May I speak with some of the other parents?

Your home-district special education department may have information about schools to consider. In addition, talk to other parents whose children have attended therapeutic schools. What are their opinions and suggestions? You're likely to hear significantly different views—one family may hate the same program that was perfect for another—and understanding why will help you identify the program that best meets the needs of your child.

## WHAT TO DO WHEN YOU HIT A ROADBLOCK

Sometimes the system works, and sometimes it doesn't. Even under ideal conditions, there's likely to be conflict.

A lot of problems can be resolved by talking things through. You find out more, the teacher or other specialist finds out more, everybody hashes out misunderstandings and discusses more options and ideas and eventually you come to an agreement, a starting point, something to try.

But sometimes disagreements can't be resolved. And sometimes the problems are more serious: The school refuses to implement the IEP. You discover that none of the promised services and supports are being provided, or only a few are, or by only one or two teachers. Things went well last year but the transition to this year turns into a nightmare. The district drags its feet on completing evaluations and the IEP. You feel pressured to take what's offered when your gut (or the evidence) tells you it isn't the right thing.

Disagreements, noncompliance, and other problems happen for many reasons, from a teacher not understanding what's expected or required to willful disregard.

Things aren't working when

- you disagree with one or more of the accommodations and want to challenge the IEP;

- the recommendations aren't being applied, regardless of the reason;

- recommendations aren't being applied consistently or correctly;

- your requests for initial evaluations, an IEP meeting, IEP review, or other meetings are denied or delayed;

- the recommendations of the IEP are being applied but aren't helping, for example, if your child is making little or no progress toward short-term objectives; comes home more frustrated, anxious, and wound up than before; starts having or has more meltdowns or rage storms after school or on the weekends; resists going to school, perhaps complaining of physical symptoms such as tummy aches and headaches; starts getting in trouble or more trouble at school; struggles even more with social relationships.

There are several ways to resolve disputes, from casual, informal approaches—which you should document in writing; just because it's informal doesn't mean you don't need an accurate record—to formal legal proceedings.

Maybe all it takes is a brief parent-teacher conference to clarify things. Some parents routinely check in with the teacher personally every few days. You might chat for a minute or two when you pick your child up from school, most days just to say hi, but other days, to touch base about strategy or how things are going in general. These brief exchanges can lay the groundwork for good, ongoing communication and are an opportunity to detect and resolve problems early on.

When there's a tougher problem—you've discovered that promised programs or services aren't being provided, for example—you need to schedule a meeting with the teacher. You want to make sure you and the teacher will have enough time to discuss the problem or concern you have, which will almost certainly be longer than a quick word or two curbside after school. This type of discussion, even though it's a scheduled meeting, is still informal, legally speaking.

If talking with the teacher doesn't solve the problem, you need to work your way up the hierarchy. Depending on how your school system is organized, the next person you contact might be the school principal, another school administrator, the special ed director, or, if the problem is still unresolved, the district superintendent. If you're not sure who to talk to, ask the staff or administrator in the school office for a copy of their procedure for informal dispute resolution. If they don't have a copy, call the district office. Don't take no for an answer; they're required by law to have this information available for the asking.

You're not required to begin with or go through the informal approach. If you've tried it before and things are the same or worse, it may be time to request mediation or to begin formal legal proceedings by requesting a *due process hearing*. It's not an either/or choice: You can begin with the informal approach, later request a due process hearing, and continue with informal settlement negotiations throughout.

Regardless of which approach you use, remember to keep written records of everything. The formal process also includes specific forms and notices that you must provide, beginning with a due process complaint notice.

The school district is also required to provide several forms to you. The *prior notice* form should include why the school is or is not doing something. The school district is legally required to send this notice to you whenever it takes or refuses to take certain actions.

The *procedural safeguards* notice tells you about your educational rights as a parent. You'll see (or should see) this notice from the very beginning: The district is required to provide it when your child is referred for his initial evaluation, as well as when you file a complaint, anytime you request the notice, and at least once a year.

The law requires that both of these notices be written clearly, in language that regular people can understand, not in dense "legalese." If you need the form in a language other than English, the school must provide either a translated version in the language you need or a translator.

If despite your best efforts, your child's school does not plan for or provide the free appropriate public education in the least restrictive environment that your child needs and is entitled to by law, you have the right to pursue legal action against the school. You probably should hire an attorney who is experienced in special education law to represent you, but you're not required by law to do so, that is, you can represent yourself. Either way, it's a good idea to talk with an attorney, an educational advocate, or both before you begin legal proceedings.

## KEEPING YOUR COOL

On the days when the bureaucracy drives you nuts, or you're trying to explain your child's disability and needs for the umpteenth time, take a deep breath and remember that what you are campaigning for is *what best meets the needs of your child*.

The school can (and often will) disagree with you about what constitutes the "least restrictive environment" and what, exactly, your child needs. Listen to what they say, but don't simply accept it as true because they say it. The school may be offering a particular accommodation or service because they are convinced it is the best of all possible solutions—or because it's what they've done before or what they always try first, or they don't know about other alternatives, or they think this will be "good enough" and it involves the least amount of money, time, and hassle for them.

You know your child better than anyone else does, and as a parent, you are an equal on the IEP team. Your thoughts and opinions carry as much weight as those of the other team members. The entire team must reach consensus. An IEP isn't approved by unanimous vote, and you can't veto it (though you can refuse services), but no one else on the team can veto it, either.

There are many right answers for every question concerning educational needs. To figure out which right answers are the best right answers at this precise time for your specific child, keep asking:

*What best meets the needs of my child?*

---

ALPHABET SOUP

The world of special education is filled with acronyms. These are some of the more common ones.

504      Refers to Section 504 of the Rehabilitation Act of 1973 and the Americans with Disabilities Act (ADA). Both address the civil rights of people who have disabilities, including guaranteeing equal access to educational services. Section 504 requires that school districts provide a free appropriate public education to children with disabilities (including bipolar and other brain disorders and learning disabilities) within the district's jurisdiction, regardless of the nature or severity of the

| | |
|---|---|
| (504 cont'd) | student's disability. Under the 504 and ADA, the school district must meet the educational needs of students with disabilities as adequately as it meets the educational needs of students who do not have disabilities. ADA expands the reach of 504 to include schools and agencies that do not receive public funding—private and parochial schools must comply with these laws even if they don't receive any federal funds. If your child has an IEP, the 504 requirements are incorporated within it. If your child doesn't have an IEP, she may still qualify for accommodations under the 504. |
| ED | Emotionally disturbed (often refers to a special classroom, the "ED class"); see also SED. |
| ESY | Extended school year. Special education and related services provided during summer vacation. Some children risk losing the benefits they've gained during the school year if they have a long break from school. These students need special education and related services through summer vacation as part of their free appropriate public education. |
| FAPE | Free appropriate public education. Providing the special education and related services that a student with disabilities needs in order to benefit from his or her education program. The services must be provided at public expense and must follow the IEP. |

IDEA     Individuals with Disabilities Education Act. The federal law that addresses education for students who need special education and related services because they have one or more disabilities (disabilities include bipolar disorder, ADHD, and learning disabilities).

IEP     Individualized educational program (also called *individualized educational plan*). The written educational plan developed by the IEP team listing the specific services the student will receive. The IEP should include the results of evaluations and testing done as part of initial and follow-up assessment (including results from independent evaluations), medical diagnoses and other relevant medical information provided by qualified healthcare professionals, measurable goals and objectives, and observations about the student's learning style and strengths.

IEP Team     The group of people who create the IEP for a student. The team includes parents, appropriate school personnel (the student's teachers, special ed teacher, other specialists), and other people who know about the student and the student's educational needs (for example, advocate, psychiatrist, or therapist).

LD     Learning disability, learning disabled (also "learning differences" or "learning different").

LRE        Least restricted environment. IDEA requires
           that students who have disabilities be edu-
           cated in regular (mainstream) classrooms
           with students who don't have disabilities to
           the maximum extent appropriate. If the IEP
           team determines that, even with supplemen-
           tary aids and services, the student's place-
           ment in the mainstream classroom won't be
           successful, the student can be placed in a spe-
           cial class or separate school.

SED        Severely emotionally disturbed (often refers
           to a special classroom, the "SED class"); see
           also ED.

SPED,      Special education. Instruction designed to
special ed  meet the unique needs of a child who has
           one or more disabilities. Special ed encom-
           passes instruction conducted in the class-
           room, home, hospitals and institutions, and
           other settings. (It includes physical educa-
           tion, too!)

Thanks to Tami Joia, president, Individual Development to Education, Attitudes, and Solutions Corporation (I.D.E.A.S.), for her work as an advocate as well as her generosity in sharing information included in this chapter; and to Marcie Lipsitt, parent and advocate, and Susan Resko, executive director, CABF, for providing suggestions and additional resources.

# Chapter 10

# DEFENDING THE CASTLE

## STRATEGIES FOR THRIVING

*On the days Michael's meds are working, he's well behaved. This is not one of those days.*

*His current eruption has left a swath of broken toys and toppled furniture. His mom, who is petite but strong, is literally sitting on him, waiting for the storm to blow itself out.*

*Over the din of Michael's shrieking and swearing, she hears the phone ring. Her older son answers it and shouts down the hall that it's Grandma. At the same time, her younger son hollers from the bathroom that he needs help with the toilet paper. After her older son brings her the cordless phone, she asks him to please help his brother in the bathroom. He stares at her for a long minute, then says, "Okay, but you owe me big-time, Mom."*

*Grandma asks how things are going. Michael's mom laughs ruefully and says, "Well, I'm sitting on Michael . . ."*

*Nathan's parents sit close together in the waiting room. They were high school sweethearts and come from big, rough-and-tumble families. Nathan was recently diagnosed with bipolar and is angry and defiant much of the time. His parents are working hard to use the parenting strategies the therapist recommends, which are a lot different from the ones they grew up with. If they'd behaved the way Nathan does when they were kids, their parents would have whomped them.*

*They are still coming to terms with the fact that Nathan's problem behaviors are symptoms of his illness, not manipulative or deliberate.*

*Alicia has two dollars in her pocket and is almost out of gas. When she pulls into the gas station, she spends the money on lottery tickets, figuring that she'll buy gas with her winnings and have plenty left over for shopping, too. But of course she doesn't win, and now she's completely broke. She pulls out of the station and drives for a while, trying to decide if she should head toward home or her friend's house, her original destination. She runs out of gas but manages to call AAA on her cell phone. The dispatcher tells her they can help, but she'll have to pay for the gas up-front. Alicia calls home and asks her brother to bring gasoline. He says no, but agrees to bring enough cash for her to pay AAA.*

There's no question that, as the parent of a child who has bipolar, you have an incredibly tough job. You need all the usual parenting skills, with extra helpings of tenacity and endurance, a thick skin, and a good sense of humor. The patience of Mother Teresa and the serenity of a Buddhist monk come in handy, too!

The home of a child or teen with bipolar disorder is often chaotic. Parents are besieged by the demands and challenges of the child who has bipolar and by the needs of their other children. Siblings are in frequent conflict with each other, their parents, and their affected brother or sister. Parents are often in conflict with each other, too, as well as exhausted, frustrated, and overwhelmed. It's hard to accept that your child is different. It's painful to watch her struggle. It can be tough to love and accept unconditionally a child who crashes through life like a hurricane, earthquake, and tsunami rolled into one. To make it through, you need effective strategies and techniques that recognize the challenges of raising a family affected by bipolar disorder.

The "job" of children is to grow and learn, becoming more responsible and confident, and eventually joining society as independent, autonomous, self-reliant adults. That's challenging for healthy children, and of course much more so for those who have bipolar.

As a parent, you have more influence over your child than anyone else, even on the days when you're convinced nothing works or ever will. The best parenting in the world won't cure your child's bipolar, but effective parenting combined with appropriate treatment will help manage his illness.

The stories and suggestions in this chapter do not soft-pedal the challenges or set up unrealistic expectations, either good or bad. They do provide ideas, strategies, and examples to help you and those around you understand, support, and accept these extraordinary young people, your child among them.

*The child you thought you had turns out to be someone different, and for a while, you think everything is terrible, because bipolar is a tough illness, and it's hard on everybody. My son didn't grow up to be a CEO like his brother. He didn't leave home at eighteen, ready to take on the world the way his younger sister did. But he did find his way in the world. Yes, he has bipolar. He also has wonderful gifts to offer.*

JJ'S MOTHER

Accepting your child for who she is, illness and neurological glitches included, begins with letting go of the "perfect child" image you carry. All parents go through this to some degree. When you fall in love with your baby, you know she's perfect. Over time, as you get to know each other, you recognize that she's thrilled to go to the zoo but doesn't like ballet class. You let go of the dream of raising a brilliant dancer and replace it with something that fits your daughter better. You might feel a little sad that you won't have a ballerina in the family after all, but a veterinarian or safari tour guide is fine, once you get used to the idea.

Parents whose children have disabilities or illnesses go through this process, too, but instead of being a slow and gradual transition, it's often sudden and jarring. One day, you're struggling to cope with your *child* and the next, you're struggling to cope with your *mentally ill child*. She's still your child, but with the diagnosis, she's something else, too.

During chaotic times, you'll be too busy dealing with the crisis of the moment to dwell on this difference. When things calm down a little, you may feel sad, panicky, or worried. You may feel even more grief-stricken during stretches of time when her bipolar symptoms are well controlled. It's during those times that other problems—plus disorders, poor social skills, cognitive problems, learning disabilities—are more obvious. You're fretting about your child—can a child like yours have a normal life, a good future?—but you're also mourning the loss of what might have been if she'd never become ill. This grieving process is normal, and allowing yourself to go through it will help you accept and attend to the needs of your child.

*Sarah reports that her son Andrew's irritability has gotten a lot worse lately. Every day from the time he gets up to the time he goes to bed is nonstop arguing, sometimes with his sister but mostly with his mom. "I'm the Wicked Witch of the West," Sarah grimaces. She's also noticed that Andrew is more disorganized and is forgetting things he usually doesn't have trouble with, like brushing his teeth. If she asks him to do something, he yells at her and then acts babyish and clingy. They're all struggling to cope with the upheaval caused by Andrew's behavior.*

*Andrew's symptom flare-up has been hard on Sarah. She's kept her equilibrium by reminding herself—and Andrew—that there's a lot going on in his life right now. He just wrapped up his science fair project, which was well done but stressful. He's getting ready to graduate from elementary school to middle school, and his two best friends are moving far away.*

*She also points out how well he's doing despite this rough patch. Some kids in his class have been picking on him and there have been a few scuffles, but Andrew kept his cool and successfully stood up for himself. He's also ridden the bus to school and back on his own most days.*

When you live every day with the chaos and upheaval of bipolar and bipolar plus, your view of your child can change in other ways, too.

It doesn't take many months of outlandish or disruptive behavior before your attention is focused on all the things that are wrong with your child. Medication, therapy, and special ed concentrate on identifying and fixing problems. Everything is about the illness and the problems it causes. In the crush of all that's wrong, it's easy to overlook your child's strengths.

Your child is not a bag of bipolar symptoms. He is a full, complete, complex human being with talents and strengths. Recognizing and helping your child recognize his strengths helps him build skills and feel competent and confident. It helps him learn how to leverage his strengths to improve weaker areas. And it helps protect the relationship between you and your child.

You want the best relationship you can have with your child. That doesn't mean you're trying to be his friend or buddy; you are still the parent. Accepting your child for who he is and facilitating his strengths doesn't mean you abdicate your responsibilities as a parent; it is, in fact, the heart of responsible parenting.

In the example above, Sarah's parenting approach does more than help herself and Andrew through the current rough patch. Through it, Andrew is learning that what's happening in his life—the stress from the science fair, the sadness of friends leaving—can affect his bipolar symptoms. He's learning that he has some great strengths even during these times. And he's learning that his mom loves and accepts him no matter what, even during the rough patches. These important lessons are forming the foundation Andrew needs to become a competent, independent adult.

*Both of Melanie's daughters have disabilities: Jenna has Down syndrome and Marissa has bipolar disorder. Melanie realized that she handled Jenna's public tantrums better than Marissa's because she knew other people saw Jenna's physical differences, which are common in Down syndrome. When Jenna had a meltdown, bystanders were sympathetic and offered assistance. But when Marissa had a meltdown, Melanie was sure onlookers thought she was a horrible parent, which filled her with shame and guilt. She recognized that her different reactions to her daughters stemmed from her worries about what onlookers thought, not from a difference in her daughters' behaviors. During future tantrums, she still felt a flash of embarrassment, but she set it aside and focused on helping Marissa de-escalate and recover.*

Your relationship with your child relies on you finding a balance between the extremes of being highly critical and being overinvolved. Some parents lean more toward the critical; they're distant, demanding, perhaps rigid or perfectionistic. Instead of focusing on their child's strengths, they zero in on anything that seems different or unacceptable no matter how minor and harangue their child about it. Other parents lean more toward the overinvolved end of the spectrum; they're extremely protective and try to do everything for their child. As with most things in life, something in between these two extremes is best.

How you view your child's illness will affect how you cope with it, which in turn will affect how the people in your child's world will respond. That includes family members as well as the general public.

Some families seem to have a knack for this. They can see the humor in less harmful behaviors, or they have no trouble matter-of-factly excusing themselves from a situation that is about to cause or has already caused a major meltdown.

For other parents, it isn't as easy. They feel embarrassed or ashamed of their ill child, worried or afraid that other people will judge them or accuse them of wrongdoing. Feeling this way doesn't make you a bad parent; it's just the way you tend to respond. Understanding why you're reacting the way you are and deliberately trying a different approach can help—and that's something all good parents do.

*Nine-year-old Samuel is normally a sweet kid, cheerful, generally helpful, rarely rude. Lately, he's been a bossy know-it-all, defiant and demanding. His symptom breakthrough was modest and intermittent at first, but now it's clear that mania is behind a lot of his behavior and attitude.*

Parents whose children have bipolar disorder learn to adjust behavior expectations according to how their children are doing. There is always a struggle between the medical reality that your child really does not have control over symptoms and the real and appropriate need for setting limits. It isn't always clear whether you're observing manipulative behavior or the symptoms of the disorder. Figuring out which is which for your child is part of the art of parenting.

When there's lots of cycling—you're adjusting meds or the meds aren't working, or it's just turned out to be a bad day—you lower your expectations of what's acceptable. That might mean your son doesn't have to do chores today or sit through dinner with the rest of the family. You ignore annoying behaviors that you might correct on better days.

To some, changing expectations seems like bad parenting. "Be consistent" is one of the most common bits of parenting advice, and generally speaking, it's good advice. Kids do need consistency—and besides, if Susie could do her chores and be civil to her little sister yesterday, she should be able to do it today, shouldn't she?

By now you know that bipolar doesn't work that way. Yesterday was a good day: Susie's moods were stable and the two of you avoided anything that might trigger problem behaviors. Today, her bipolar brain isn't working the same way. Her moods are spinning nonstop, everything's a trigger, she's had twenty-two tantrums in the last hour, and you've reached the point where you're seriously considering duct-taping her to the kitchen chair. Insisting that she perform up to yesterday's expectations isn't going to help, and it isn't something she can do anyway.

These are the times when you tell her you know she's going through a hard time and that you will help her get through it.

As she gets healthier and her mood stabilizes, you raise the expectations again, without expecting perfection or complete consistency.

There may be times when you feel as if you're continually lowering your expectations for your child. You worry that she'll never be able to achieve anything, or worse, that she'll learn that all she has to do to dodge responsibility is to act up. Experience and research both say otherwise.

Adjusting your expectations doesn't mean you're giving in or giving up. It means that you are meeting your child where he is—accepting what he's capable of right now, at this moment—and moving on from there.

You may also need to adjust your expectations if you're basing those expectations on how old your child is.

Children and teens with bipolar often have delays in emotional development and lag behind their age-mates in social skills. That's because they're not learning at the same rate. Their bipolar symptoms interfere with their ability to experience people and surroundings the way other kids do. Even when their symptoms are stabilized, children with bipolar don't know how to interact as well; they simply haven't had the same practice with day-to-day social interactions as other children.

When your child's mood is stabilized, you can work on overcoming these delays through a combination of approaches, including social skills groups, where your child learns and practices the skills; role playing, which is one-on-one therapy to learn and practice age-appropriate behavior; and group therapy, including anger management classes.

*Matt is in junior high; little brother Corey is in first grade; and Michael, who has bipolar, is in the middle.*

*Matt says it's really hard and sometimes embarrassing to have a brother like Michael. He knows why the consequences for his misbehavior are different from Michael's—he's not allowed to swear at all, for example—but it bugs him. Corey says that sometimes Michael's really mean and tries to hurt him. When Matt points out that Corey loves to "poke the hornets' nest," doing stuff Corey knows will set Michael off, Corey grins and says that Matt is his best defender.*

*It isn't all bad; the brothers agree that Michael is funny and sometimes nice. Matt knows he'll help Michael if he needs help when they get older.*

*Michael is glad that he has brothers even though he knows that their teasing is one of his triggers. Matt is really growing up, he says, so it's nice to have a little brother who will still play and have fun with you. Having a big brother who's close in age (Matt's just two years older than Michael) is good, too, because he can talk to him about things, like what to expect when he starts middle school next year.*

*The boys' mother, Emma, says discipline for the three is a big problem because the rules have to be different for each of them. That would be true to a certain extent because of their ages—expectations for a six-year-old should be different from those for a thirteen-year-old—but Emma's learned to adjust expectations for Michael based on his symptoms. She doesn't argue when Matt and Corey complain that it's unfair. Of course it's unfair—but that does not change the fact that they are responsible for following the rules that apply to them.*

Raising a child who has bipolar is hard on everyone. The stress affects the entire family, including your other children. The behaviors and problems of bipolar magnify normal sibling rivalry and routinely disrupt everything. It isn't unusual for siblings to hate their affected brother or sister. Even if they're old enough to understand that an illness is behind the problems, it doesn't change the fact that their brother or sister makes life miserable. In addition to talking with your children about the affected child's illness, acknowledge how difficult it

is for the siblings. Encourage them to pursue their own interests and develop friendships. Participating in sibling support
groups and therapy (family, siblings-only, or individual) can
be helpful, too.

*Aaron's dad has explained to his son umpteen times the connection be-
tween his illness, the meds, and his behavior, but he still doesn't get it.
They both agree that he had lots of ups and downs for a while and that
things are better now. Aaron is sure that the problems were caused by
the situation "back then," when his older brother was running with a
bad crowd, which worried and frightened Aaron. So if he does have
bipolar (he's willing to allow for the possibility but isn't entirely convinced), it was the combination of the situation and the illness that
made him "flip out" all the time. Now that the situation is better, Aaron
wants to decrease or stop taking his meds. He thinks that if he works
harder, he'll do okay.*

*Rita is having a similar problem with her seventeen-year-old
daughter, Taryn. Taryn had been stable for a while and decided to decrease, then stop, taking her meds. Without meds, she shifted into hypomania and felt great—better than great. Rita knew they were headed
for trouble but had a hard time convincing Taryn that she needed to
restart treatment with meds. Taryn was angry and suspicious, and de-
manded to know why her mother wanted to make her do something that
would take away the happiness she felt.*

*Aaron understands that one of the conditions of living at home
and getting his driver's license is taking his meds. During therapy sessions, the therapist spends time helping Aaron think through why his
dad emphasizes meds. At home, Aaron's dad encourages him to read
about what life is like with and without meds for other people who have
mood disorders.\* He's also encouraging Aaron to keep a log of his
moods to see if it helps him recognize that his ups and downs occur in a
variety of situations.*

\*For example, see "Depression and Bipolar Support Alliance" and other re-
sources listed in Appendix E.

*Taryn is tugging hard at Rita's apron strings. She's in a hurry to be on her own—a combination of being seventeen and grandiosity-fueled overconfidence. Requiring her to stick with treatment in order to live at home isn't going to motivate her to take her meds.*

*Taryn has her sights set on the arts and drama department of a small private college. Rita suspects that if Taryn's bipolar is under control, she can do well there. Taking her meds and going to therapy become conditions Taryn must meet if she wants her parents to pay for college.*

Bipolar disorder brings with it a lack of insight, which makes it even tougher to raise your child. It's difficult, sometimes impossible, for children and adults who have bipolar to understand and accept the impact of the illness on themselves. Lack of insight is a big reason why some children, especially teens, pressure their parents to let them stop taking their meds. You may need to leverage other things your child wants to ensure that he'll stick with his treatment.

Showing your child or teen the evidence of how changes in treatment have been reflected in changes in behavior can help reassure her that you're doing the right thing and that the treatment really is making a difference. Continue to guide and educate her (which is not the same as nagging!) about lifestyle issues, including medication and other treatment, that are central to managing her illness.

*Kevin is full of swagger and bravado; he just celebrated his eighteenth birthday. His psychiatrist goes through his new rights of confidentiality with him. Kevin gleefully announces that he's quitting meds and probably won't come back for another appointment. He's going on a road trip, it's all set; he's leaving the day after graduation.*

*His parents are frantic with worry. Kevin's already been in trouble with the law, and they know he's flunking several of his courses. They discuss their options with the psychiatrist and plan a variety of strategies to negotiate the rocky terrain ahead.*

Older children with bipolar may use poor judgment about relationships and get into risky or inappropriate situations. Severe behavior problems resulting from bipolar may have increasingly serious consequences, which accelerate rapidly as the child reaches the age of majority—for example, criminal actions during mania can result in increasingly severe legal problems.

When your child reaches the magic age of eighteen, all the rules change. Your mostly grown child now has the right to make his or her own decisions, including the decision to keep mental health information confidential—even from you, and even if you're paying the bills. Insurance, treatment, and confidentiality issues are more complicated. Your carefully assembled treatment team may no longer be able to discuss your child's situation with you—or each other—unless your child consents. Yet you know that your child isn't ready for the independence and responsibility of true adulthood.

Parents often feel powerless at this stage of their child's life. Other kids this age, including perhaps brothers and sisters, are going off to college, beginning to live independently, finding fulfilling work—in short, becoming productive members of society—and parents worry whether their child with bipolar will be able to join their ranks.

Many teens with bipolar disorder do succeed in school and go on to college. They find fulfilling work and make positive contributions to society. They find their place in the world; they just need specialized help to achieve these normal milestones.

*Meds, therapy, school, special programs, setting limits, tracking symptoms, figuring out what to do next. Every time I read another article or listen to the news or find a new Web site, I wonder what else should be on my to-do list. Do I need to add "check backpack for firearms" or "review essays for signs of suicidal thoughts"? How about, "do personal self-checks hourly to determine whether I'm in denial about his abilities— or mine. If the answer is no, continue with this list. If the answer is yes, go to sublist A and find a therapist, a parenting class, a different school, new meds."*

*The pressure to put the "right things" on the list never lets up. And once I've got the list, I still have to decide which of those "right things" are important enough to do right now, because the one thing that's always true is that there is never enough time and money to do everything.*

*My friends who've already been through this with their kids tell me that I'll never get everything on the list done, and that the best any of us can hope for at the end of the day, when we send our children off into the world, is that we'll have done enough of the right things on the list. Not all, just enough.*

JUDY, PARENT

In our drive to help our children, we want to fix everything right now, but bipolar and the plus disorders cause so many problems that it's easy to feel overwhelmed. You and your child will have a better shot at success if you create a list of the behaviors you want to change and rank them by how important each one is to you. What worries or aggravates you the most? Causes the most difficulty for your child or your family? Will make the fastest or biggest difference if it's improved?

There's no right or wrong way to make your list. The highest priority problem on the list is the problem that is most important to you, and it's the place to begin.

Your list isn't carved in stone. When things change—a new problem crops up or an old one is no longer a problem—your list changes, too.

*Jonathon has done a slow burn all day about his "stupid" video game controller, punctuated by explosions when his mom tells him (again and again, because he won't stop asking) that no, she won't buy him another one, the one he has works just fine. In addition to the severe irritability common in mania, Jonathon's also stuck in "mission mode," focused on getting a game controller and unable to shift his attention to anything else.*

Huge reactions to small triggers are a common problem in pe-diatric bipolar. Confrontations, explosive outbursts, conflict, and defiance overrun our best attempts at calm and peaceful parenting.

What are your child's triggers? Where is he most likely to encounter problems? Grocery store, shopping mall, anyplace with noisy crowds? Waiting for the bus before school, espe-cially when he hasn't had a good night's sleep? Anytime he's asked to do a chore or his homework?

Although the specific triggers may be unique to your child, out-of-proportion reactions, including rage storms, connect them to the symptoms of bipolar.

The first choice in dealing with triggers is to avoid them altogether, but this isn't always possible. And there are situa-tions where some days, your child is fine, or fine for a while, and other days when chaos reigns no matter what you do. Your task as a parent is learning to recognize your child's trig-gers, avoid them when possible, and make a graceful exit be-fore problem behaviors escalate.

If the grocery store is an invitation for disaster, find a way to do grocery shopping when you don't have to take your child with you: during school, when Grandma can babysit, or when Dad is home. Order your groceries online or over the phone and have them delivered, or call out for pizza.

If your child announces that "It's time to go *now*," then it's time to go, even if everything seems fine.

If his behavior is getting a little ragged or you have a gut feeling that something's amiss, it's time to go, even if no one else thinks anything is wrong.

Preventing a meltdown or rage storm whenever possible is the best approach. Some families use a code word or phrase to indicate that the child has reached his limit and needs to leave.

"Sorry, we have to go, Bobby isn't feeling well and is hav-ing a tough time" should be delivered with the same straight-forward tone, concern, and confidence as if Bobby had asthma and you were telling bystanders he was having an asthma attack.

These parenting strategies do not mean you are "giving in" or letting your child "run your life." By avoiding triggers and leaving situations that your child cannot handle as soon as problems arise, you're providing your child with an alternative and safe environment. You're also helping her recognize when she's revving up on her way to an outburst. This awareness gives her the ability to make choices.

If she can recognize the feeling of "I might lose control," she will have the ability at that moment to choose from several strategies that she's learned. For example, she can remove herself from the situation, or she can use a coping strategy to deal with the situation, handling it differently from previous times.

When you respect your child's request to leave a setting now, you're acknowledging his ability to recognize for himself that the situation is about to pass the level he can handle. You're respecting his ability to take appropriate action that prevents inappropriate behavior.

---

Research shows that yelling at a raging child or teen INCREASES the rage and makes it harder for the child to calm down. The more you shout, the worse it gets.

To help your child calm down:

- Don't shout.
- Be calm (or act as if you are).
- Lower your voice. Use soothing tones. Speak quietly (or not at all).

---

*Katie hates everything about school except for her art and drama teacher, because her teacher understands and encourages her. The teacher isn't bothered by anime-pink hair or unusual clothing combinations.*

She views Katie's unique sense of style and flair for the dramatic as strengths, outward signs of intelligence and creativity.

Katie's parents are divorced and share custody. Her mother frequently complains about Katie's hair and clothing. Most of her interactions with Katie begin with lectures and harsh criticism and, not surprisingly, turn into arguments and shouting matches.

Katie's father and stepmother are more supportive of Katie. They provide a welcoming environment that nurtures Katie's strengths, offers opportunities for her to build skills, and keeps disruptions to a minimum.

There are many reasons why Katie's mom might be so critical. She might be worried about her daughter, or have strong beliefs about what's acceptable attire, or be treating her daughter the same way her own parents treated her when she was growing up, assuming that since it worked for her, it will work for Katie, too.

But Katie's behaviors and mood are worse, not better, when she's with her mother. They're both miserable, and the quality of their relationship continues to deteriorate.

It's a different story when Katie's with her dad or stepmom. Her behavior and moods are in better control. She's more confident. It's clear that the relationship is positive on both sides. When she hits a rough patch, she recovers more quickly.

Katie's mom isn't necessarily a bad mom, but the parenting style she's using, regardless of why, isn't working with Katie. To be the parent Katie needs, Mom will have to expand her repertoire, learning and using parenting techniques that focus less on being the ruling authority and more on being a listener and facilitator.


Terry was rebellious to begin with, and when he was about fifteen, it got worse. One of the ways it showed up was in his physical appearance. He would dress up in all kinds of costumes. There was a goth phase, a ratty clothes phase, several months when he refused to use soap or deodorant because they weren't "natural." He even wore fake fingernails and his sister's glitter T-shirts for a while.

*His mom realized that most of this behavior was Terry trying to provoke her, to see if she'd love and accept him no matter what. She knew the behavior itself wasn't dangerous, so she did her best to roll with it, and she tried to protect him from the worst of the harassment she knew he'd get at school. If Terry's behavior had included signs of hypersexuality or breaks with reality (he didn't just dress like a pirate, but thought he was a pirate), her response would have been different: an appointment with Terry's doctor to discuss bipolar symptoms resurfacing.*

Are *you* a trigger? Many children and teens with bipolar are more rebellious by nature. Authority figures, including parents, and the command "no" are common triggers for meltdowns and outbursts at any age. The harder you try to make your child into something he's not, the more resistance you'll get. Conformity is not going to happen with these kids.

As the parent, you control how you approach these situations. You can criticize, confront, or demand that she do it your way this instant. Or, you can keep the communication open, ask your teen to help you understand what's going on, and use that information as you guide your child in ways that enable her to broaden her strengths and skills.

Part of normal teen development is self-expression that announces to the world, "I'm not a little kid and I'm not my parents, either!" Teens who have bipolar are often more over the top in expressing their individuality. You'll have to use every ounce of your support, love, and communication skills, not to mention patience, to get them through the turbulence. You may need to enlist the support of a therapist who's experienced with both bipolar and adolescence, especially if conflicts continue to escalate.

---

### AVOIDING "NO"

"No" is a wonderful word: short, direct, to the point. Unfortunately, it's also a significant trigger for many children and teens with bipolar. Instead of saying no, try redirecting or reframing. Suppose your daughter wants to go out with friends on a school night, something she's not allowed to do. Tell her no and she's likely to erupt in a rage. On the other hand, if you remind her that she and her friends will be getting together Friday and ask her what they're planning to do, maybe comment on how anticipating Friday's outing will make it even more fun, or suggest an alternate activity for tonight such as calling a friend to discuss Friday's plans, there's a better chance that she'll maintain self-control. Collaborative problem solving (Chapter 8) can be an effective method to manage situations ahead of time and maneuver through them when they occur, all without using "no."

---

*Keisha hates homework. She's exhausted from holding it together at school all day and refuses to do homework unless she gets a break first. Her mom points out that Keisha's "breaks" last until bedtime and that she's never too tired to play video games or talk with her friends on the phone.*

*They're both right. They agree that Keisha will have "decompression time" until suppertime. After supper, she has half an hour to settle into "homework mode," and then she will do her homework. She's responsible for setting the timer for thirty minutes. She should be able to finish her homework in an hour (something that's specified on her IEP), which leaves enough time to do other quiet activities before bedtime. Keisha agrees to "no complaining or arguing when it's time to shift to homework." Her mother agrees to "no nagging Keisha to get started," which they define as no more than three reminders. If Keisha doesn't fulfill her end of the bargain, she'll lose phone privileges for that evening and the next day's decompression time.*

You tell your daughter it's time to start her homework. She says later; when "later" rolls around, she says she can't because she's too tired.

You ask your son to clean his room like he promised. He tells you to get off his case, he'll do it when he wants to and not when you tell him. Two days later, the room is still a mess.

There's more to these conflicts than parent-teen power struggles.

Kids with bipolar generally don't have a good time sense. They'll agree to do something, know they need to do it, then fritter away the time during which they should have done it. They'll rebel against your request that a task be done immediately, refusing to comply unless they can do it on their own timeline, which gets reset to zero every time you remind them. This is especially noticeable in teens because we expect teens to be better at time management than younger children are.

Engaging your teen in the decisions surrounding homework, chores, and other responsibilities may improve the situation.

Together, you decide what has to be done, what the constraints are, and what the consequences are if the task isn't completed as agreed. In short, you make a contract with your teen. It's often a good idea to put the agreement in writing because when it comes time to comply, some kids will be furious and claim that they never agreed to the plan. A written plan helps prevent miscommunication and disagreements. You'll both be able to refer to the written agreement and avoid emotional landmines that could trigger a rage storm.

Here's another example.

Nathan has to do his own laundry as well as several other routine chores, and laundry has become a major trigger. He comes home, his mom tells him to do his laundry, and he erupts in rage.

When his therapist asked Nathan if he minded doing laundry, Nathan said no, he just didn't want to do it right then. They talked about ways to solve the problem, including what consequences Nathan should get if he didn't do this chore. Then he, his parents, and the therapist wrote down the agreement: Nathan would have twenty-four hours to do his laundry. If he didn't do it within the allotted time, he wouldn't be allowed to use the computer for one day. The consequence was important enough to matter to him, but not so severe as to be unfair. Nathan could accept this consequence without having a meltdown because he was involved in the decision-making process.

The contract worked quite well for the first week or so. In fact, it worked so well that Nathan's dad began to press for "improvements." When Nathan was playing video games, his dad would say, "Why don't you go start your laundry now?" Nathan would say, "No, I have twenty-four hours," and things would escalate from there.

Nathan's dad was angry and frustrated; he was just trying to teach Nathan some organization. Nathan was defiant and oppositional; Dad wasn't keeping the deal.

With the therapist's help, they reworked the contract. Nathan, suspicious that his parents would try to add things later, wanted to include his other routine chores. The new version also includes requirements for respectful behaviors for and from everyone and specific actions Nathan will take when he starts to get angry. They also discussed the consequences of not complying and wrote those into the contract so there wouldn't be any surprises.

The end result is a contract that helps Nathan do his chores with minimal disruption and gives him specific steps to follow when he escalates. The contract also helps his parents use a less confrontational approach, which for Nathan is more effective than the more authoritarian style they were used to.

CONTRACT FOR NATHAN AND HIS PARENTS

Nathan will:

1. Make bed in morning; empty dishes when asked; clean up after self before leaving the room.

2. Work on organization and time management for laundry and trash.

3. Nathan has twenty-four hours to complete all chores except for those listed in #1 above.

4. When Nathan is escalating, he will say, "I can't talk about this right now." Within twenty-four to forty-eight hours, when he is calm, he and one or both parents will sit down together to problem solve. Plan: Identify the problem, keep the emotion out of it, calmly discuss the problem (or event, for example, swearing at Mom) that was unacceptable, discuss the consequences for action (example: no computer).

5. Avoid power struggles; don't raise voice or swear; don't make faces, roll eyes, or use sarcasm; be respectful.

6. Consequences for not completing daily chores: no cell phone for one day plus chore has to be done; for other chores: no computer for one day.

Contracts and good faith negotiations can be powerful tools when moods are stable. If your child's symptoms flare up, you may need to put the contract on hold until he's able to try again.

### My child holds it together at school; why can't she cope at home?

Part of the reason is that kids work so hard to be okay at school that they have nothing left to work with when they return to the safety of home. And they know how tough it will be at school, so mornings are often as difficult as the after-school crash. It's like having a bad day at work. Even without a mood disorder, if you have a lousy day on the job, you manage yourself because there will be serious social consequences if you don't. When you get home, you might yell or swear or bang the pots and pans around while preparing supper.

There's another intriguing piece to this okay-at-school puzzle.

The kind of thinking you do at school (or work) is different from the kind of thinking you do at home. Different kinds of thinking engage different areas of your brain. Shifting to a new area can derail whatever the first area was doing. For example, if you're about to cry and you start to count, you'll derail the crying. Counting to ten when you're angry helps in part because you stop what you're doing long enough to count; it also helps because your brain can't count (a cognitive function) and be angry (an emotional function) at the same time. Most of this brain-area shifting goes on without our being consciously aware of it. We find ways to distance or distract ourselves from our emotions until we're in a place where we know it's okay to let them out.

It's possible that the demands for cognitive thinking at school keep your child's moodiness at bay. When he comes home, his brain shifts away from the cognitive areas to those that control emotions and moods.

Regardless of the reason, it's important to remember that kids who have bipolar need downtime after school or other intense activities. As mentioned earlier, insisting that homework or chores be done as soon as they get home is unrealistic.

*Jeff was geeky and quiet until puberty, when practically overnight he turned into "Mr. Bravado": not quiet, not inhibited, and definitely hypersexual. His conversation is filled with sexual references. He talks about doing weird things to his genitals. His folks discovered him surfing the Internet for porn. A little checking revealed that he'd accessed an incredible number of sites, including many with extreme or aberrant content. He bragged about going online after his parents were asleep and surfing all night.*

*Steve's dad likes porn and he shares his magazines and videos with Steve. Steve was caught using the computer in the high school library to visit porn sites. The girl who complained said Steve grabbed her and made sexual comments, which he denied. He was arrested and charged with sexual assault. Because some of the sites he visited included child pornography, Steve is now required to register as a sex offender.*

Exposing children to porn is not the same as providing them straightforward information about human sexuality. We usually think of pornography as something for older people—grown-ups—like alcohol or smoking, which they can choose to either indulge in or decline. Adults generally have the cognitive ability to put these materials into context; kids don't. Parents must establish limits on materials their children and teens are not developmentally ready for. This is especially true for kids who have bipolar, because these materials can fuel hypersexuality.

Your child needs *sexual education and information,* delivered in language appropriate to your child's age and ability to understand, in a context that she can apply now. For example, telling your six-year-old, "Sex involves two people who love each other and are grown-ups" helps her understand why she shouldn't do "sex play" with her friends and the importance of boundaries ("good touch" versus "bad touch") and safety. Children who have bipolar may try to ferret out this information at an earlier age than their non-bipolar peers, which only increases the importance of being aware and keeping the lines of communication open.

*Tony doesn't have an eating disorder or body image problem; he's just hungry all the time. His parents work hard at setting and enforcing the limits that Tony needs, but when it comes to food, they often relent. The battle over food doesn't seem worth the effort, especially when they have to be so strict about everything else.*

*Although she wasn't diagnosed with bipolar until she was almost eleven, Keri has had problems with her mood for as long as she and her mom can remember. Physical activity, especially gymnastics, has always been an important part of her life and an important part of helping her moods.*

*She's been a gymnast since early grade school. She loved everything about the sport: the gym, the hours of practice, the competition. She had reached the elite ranks when she developed bipolar.*

*Several things happened in quick succession: She was too ill to continue her gymnastics and had to drop her intense workouts. She had to come to terms with a new identity of herself as a person who wasn't a top-ranked athlete. The meds she began for her treatment caused a significant and rapid weight gain. She was also lethargic, which might have been another side effect of her meds or a symptom of her bipolar, and felt too tired to do anything. And she was hungry all the time. Keri remembers waking up in the middle of the night to raid the kitchen, eating without thinking. Body image and disordered eating became difficult problems for her.*

*Keri says she didn't have body image problems when she was a little girl, but she remembers that when she was about ten years old, she ate two pieces of licorice and a few M&M's and thought, "Oh, I am so fat." It's the first time she remembers thinking of herself that way, despite the emphasis on weight and body image common in elite gymnastics. Body image and disordered eating continue to be tough challenges for her even though her weight, fitness level, and bipolar symptoms continue to improve.*

*Keri's bipolar disorder didn't cause her body image and eating difficulties, though her bipolar symptoms combined with side effects from medication (weight gain, lethargy, overeating) certainly could have contributed to its development.*

*Annamarie was diagnosed with ADHD in second grade, and*

*rediagnosed with bipolar plus ADHD in fifth grade. Even though her moods are fairly stable, she hates going to bed on time. Soccer practice used to help, but this year, practice is later in the day and bedtime is getting to be a major problem.*

In Chapter 3, we talked about changes in the circadian rhythm and the importance of good sleep hygiene in managing bipolar disorder. Sleep hygiene is part of a larger picture we call *life hygiene*. Life hygiene includes daily routines, good nutrition, physical activity, and consistent times for sleeping, waking, and eating.

The structure and healthy habits of good life hygiene are beneficial to anyone, not just kids who have bipolar. But for these kids, life hygiene is extremely important and often difficult to maintain.

Bipolar knocks your child's circadian rhythm out of whack, which causes disrupted sleep patterns. Disrupted sleep patterns—too much or too little sleep—can aggravate the bipolar symptoms. For example, sleep deprivation is both a symptom and a cause of mania: Not needing much sleep is a symptom, and not getting enough sleep can trigger or worsen it.

Light is the primary stimulus that affects our circadian rhythms, but it isn't the only one. Physical activity, eating, and social routines also influence circadian rhythms—and bipolar affects all of them, and is in turn affected by them.

Compounding the challenge of this bipolar-life hygiene interaction is the bipolar treatment itself. Some of the most effective medications commonly have overeating, carbohydrate cravings, weight gain, and lethargy as side effects. Your child may not feel full even after eating a lot of food. Add in the "risks" of our modern lifestyle—TV and video games instead of playing outside, high calorie convenience foods—and ensuring that children practice good life hygiene becomes one of our bigger challenges.

Establishing appropriate limits and encouraging healthy

dietary habits is particularly difficult for kids with bipolar. Food is a major issue for many of them. On top of the meds effect, kids with bipolar are impulsive and generally not good at delaying gratification, so it's extra hard for them to resist the urge to eat or binge. Some also use food as a coping mechanism, eating to comfort themselves when they're feeling sad or down. We don't know if kids with bipolar are more likely to develop eating disorders, but we do know that the weight gain associated with meds can trigger disordered eating and body image problems.

Food is often a big trigger for kids with bipolar. They feel hungry or have intense cravings for junk food; parents try to set limits such as healthy meals and snacks at appropriate times and in appropriate quantities, no purging or bingeing, and no excessive exercise, and chaos ensues. Some parents refuse to have sweets, fattening foods, or low-nutrition carbohydrates in the house, so their children don't have access to these kinds of foods. This can be hard on siblings who want an occasional snack or who are thin and could really use the extra calories. Some parents lock the cabinets and refrigerator.

To help your child build and maintain good life hygiene habits, focus on his strengths and interests. Encourage him to participate in physical activities he enjoys, from swimming to organized sports to Dance Dance Revolution. Don't rely on the school's gym class; many children with bipolar have a hard time coping in traditional phys ed.* You may need to add a dietician, nutritionist, endocrinologist, or therapist to your treatment team to help guide you and your child.

---

*Physical education is part of a free appropriate public education. If regular gym class isn't appropriate for your child or teen, the IEP should include an appropriate alternative: martial arts classes, dance or swim lessons, one-on-one work with a coach or personal trainer, etc.

## FROM MOMS AND DADS, TO YOU

*The pressure and stress of raising a child with such a challenging illness can push parents into opposing corners. Dads often think, "She won't set limits, so I have to." Moms think, "He's so harsh, I have to be extra loving and protective." Both parents want what's best for the child, but they're reacting to each other, trying to compensate for what each believes is a weakness in the other.*

*If you're involved in the life of your child, whether you and the other parent are together or not, your child will do much better if the two of you are on the same page when it comes to parenting decisions. That doesn't mean you always have to agree with each other or have identical parenting styles. It does mean you must support each other and present a unified front. If you're having difficulty communicating or you can't resolve disagreements about treatment or other issues, consider couples therapy or family counseling.*

*We talk with parents like you every day, parents who are resourceful and creative, who humble us with their grit and determination. Here are some of the things they tell us.*

### *From Dave:*

It's pretty hard, frustrating, to be a father. You come home at the end of the day, you're tired, and the last thing you want to deal with is a kid who's "amped up." Kids cycle really fast, and it takes a lot of patience trying to referee all day long. My wife has much more patience because she's around him more. She gets frustrated with me because I get mad at Michael in ten minutes—faster if he attacks his little brother.

Other things are hard, too, not just the behavior. We don't do stuff as a family very often because the risk of an explosion is too big. It's tough to teach his brothers not to goad him. There's a risk of real danger, and Michael's aware of that, when he's not cycling. My wife and I use a divide and conquer strategy, one parent with Michael, the other with his brothers.

I think about the future: What will happen when he gets

older, how will he be able to cope? Bipolar kids aren't inherently bad kids, but you've got to be prepared for a lot of peaks and valleys. You know he's a good kid, he means well, but when he gets in a rage, he goes after anyone nearby; it's like a switch thrown on. So I work on separating what he's experiencing—it isn't really Michael, it's the bipolar disease acting out—and it's tough because he cycles so fast. We have to be careful, on watch all the time. I know he's got this disease and he needs help coping with it for life, but I think he can do very well.

We talk to him about his illness. He's very aware, a caring and thoughtful kid, when he's not cycling. He knows he can't drink or do drugs.

When your kid is yelling or mouthing back at you, it's hard to stay calm, but if you yell, it makes it worse. It's like fanning a fire. It doesn't help to go to his level, but it's really difficult to not react to it.

Having a kid with this illness can be very destructive to your relationship. My biggest advice for other dads is to be united with your wife in terms of how you discipline and deal with everything. It doesn't help if my wife is able to control herself with Michael and I'm flying off the handle. I think dads have more problems with this. Back when I was yelling at Michael all the time, my wife said she couldn't handle it—I was putting a huge strain on her and the family, making the situation worse. Family therapy helped with that, helped us communicate better.

You have to use patience, not explode, not react. Go with your wife to therapy sessions and doctor appointments whenever you can, so you'll understand how the disease works.

### From Scott:

I had an extremely difficult time accepting that anything was wrong. Part of that was not wanting to accept my own family history. Looking back, I'm pretty sure my mother had OCD and I know my dad had terrible alcoholism. I did okay myself as a kid, and I have a grown son from a previous marriage who's fine.

All three of our boys have bipolar. It was clear from the start that something wasn't quite right with Jamie. For a long time, I kept thinking, "This isn't happening." Finally, I began to accept it in Jamie and was sure it couldn't be true of Rob. It was even worse with Daniel, because we'd perceived him as normal for so long.

I'm most successful as a parent when I engage them physically. For the two younger ones, that's sports and other physical activities, that's where we're most able to control and enjoy their environment. With Jamie, it works better to go to the museum with him. He and I are both museum-oriented people.

I work long hours because of the demands of my job, not because of the kids. My wife and I are both child-oriented and believe it's important to engage and interact with our kids, and we spend a lot of time with them. It is easier to be at work than at home. I tend to tune out or let it go until things reach a breaking point and then intervene by yelling. That's not the best way to handle things, and I'm learning to mediate. I'm working on how to do better.

It's been interesting to me to examine my family history and hear family members talk about issues that wouldn't have been discussed before—dealing with anger and explosive outbursts, the alcoholism issue, to see these in a genetic context. Some of these issues are neurological and genetic, and now there are ways to get help instead of just drinking them away. It's good to come to an understanding of why we are the way we are.

My number-one advice to other dads is to listen to your wife. My experience is that men are a lot less likely to accept the diagnosis. The moms are a lot more understanding and want to get help—and the moms get blamed for everything.

Listen to your spouse in a larger sense, too. A lot of

marriages collapse under the weight of these kids. If the husband feels left out, he tunes out and leaves. It is easier to tune out, go to work, and let the mom deal with it, but your marriage suffers. In our situation, even though we guard against it, it still tends to happen. When you're engaged, listening, actively involved, you can save your marriage.

One of the most important things for me is to appreciate the many sides of my kids and what wonderful kids they are on so many levels, not just focus on the negatives. I strive to nurture who they are, instead of having negative expectations of them.

### From Evelyn:

Learn to meditate—yoga and meditation have been lifesavers for me. Bike riding helps, too—anything that takes you into that meditative state, the "now" without being attached. Every minute of training, whether it was something I learned in a class or figured out on my own, that helped me remain calm and realize that "my kid is not me" has been important.

It's especially tough as a single mom. I am the only one taking care of her, providing for her. You have to recognize your own motivations and do whatever is necessary to keep those clean, to keep the boundaries clear. I learned that there's a difference between acting out of responsibility and acting out of duty; if you think it's your duty, then everything gets tinged with overtones that are counterproductive. Resentment creeps in.

It isn't selfish to remember that you have your own life. The things that let me have time to myself—even a few seconds—have been my salvation. It was better when I could do things that moved me in the direction I want my life to go, painting and learning to draw, for instance, but five minutes knitting in the car with the windows up and the doors locked or leafing through pattern books at the fabric store helped, too. What you do for that self-time can change. What's crucial is that you have the self-time.

### From Amelia:

Taking care of school and health issues and the unpredictable nature of [my children's] illnesses has made it really difficult to work—something which middle-class women often approach from the perspective of exhaustion or self-fulfillment. But there are much bigger issues at stake—in order to force the school to step up to the plate, we needed an advocate, then a lawyer; in order to get a lawyer, we needed money; but we have no money because I had to give up my work in order to take care of the boys. And you know if I didn't take the steps I did, the children would be in much worse shape and that would be blamed on parenting! This is all frustrating personally, since I spent six years in graduate school and would like to use my training, but it is also terrifying and depressing to have no money. It also seems to legitimize the tendency people in power have to blame the victim—poor people having less value, mental illness as a disease of the poor, etc. But the relationship is backward—poverty is a result, not a cause...
We have been really lucky because we've been able to make it work and we live a nice enough life, but it is all very precarious and we don't know how long the little pieces we have patched together will hold. We have been reduced to simply taking care of our immediate needs, relying on public health insurance, and in the process been demoted out of middle class-ness or the professional class and into the working poor.

### From Cynthia:

I really think moms get it the worst. It's a lot tougher on the moms than the dads, mainly because we are the ones setting the limits on the kids. It took me a long time to learn to draw the line, which I have to do even if it means going to the hospital. That's a tough call to make, but we decided zero tolerance on any kind of violence, because if you accept it a little, it just gets worse; it becomes routine instead of the exception.

It's more than just avoiding getting sucked into an argument. I have to really watch my tone, my word choice. I absolutely cannot argue; I must consciously, deliberately disengage. Sometimes I get in the car and drive away! Generally, it isn't that dramatic—I mostly redirect him to something that will get his mind off of whatever the problem is, maybe put a favorite movie on. He wants to start a fight—he'll follow me around, trying to draw me into an argument and actually poke me, so I have to physically disengage, sometimes physically remove myself, maybe locking myself in my room. Sometimes, my husband and I "tag-team" and I hand him off to his dad.

Figuring out how to enforce limits has been tough. When he was younger, we couldn't make him do time-outs. Now, he doesn't have to do time-outs right away, but he doesn't get anything he wants—a snack or his supper, for example—until after he's done the time-out. The rule is that he gets five minutes for every act of aggression, so some days, he could rack up an hour or more of time-out. We'll knock five minutes off if he begins his time-out right away. I also remind him that he doesn't like time-outs, which sometimes helps him stay in control.

It's a wonder I'm still married. We've gone through some horrible times. There's been a lot of "you're not handling this right" on both sides. I've battled it out with my husband, but we try. We set aside an hour every day and do something together. While our son watches a movie, we retreat to a locked room and play cards or do a crossword puzzle. It sounds simple, but it's really helped. It's a break from the stress, a time when we focus only on each other and we don't worry or talk about bipolar. You have to find a way to do this, because if you don't, it can consume your life.

When our son was in the hospital for the first time, it took us a full week to understand how much pressure we'd been under. Since then, we pay more attention to giving each other breaks intentionally, and we try to get outside for physical activity several times a week. I do yoga twice a week—it has saved my life!—and my husband does it once in a while, too, but he prefers more aerobic activity, like Rollerblading.

We use doctors and therapists and other help. We are finally understanding that this illness is a family issue, a family problem, and treatment must address the whole family. We work hard at being conscious of the value of our relationship as husband and wife, fighting for our relationship the same way we're fighting for the health of our child.

*Be confident in your ability to raise your child. You, like these parents and others, do have what it takes to be the parent your child needs.*

# Chapter 11

# SHOCK WAVE

## COPING WITH DANGER AND CRISIS

*The house is one of the biggest in town, big enough to hold the enormous Christmas tree—a fifteen-footer at least—with room to spare.*

*At the moment, however, the tree is not upright and beautiful, surrounded by a happy family celebrating the holidays in peace and harmony. It is lying on its side, lights and decorations tangled, broken, and scattered. A few gifts are under the fallen tree; most have been ripped open and thrown across the room. Furniture has been upended. Broken glass glitters on the carpet near a fallen lamp.*

*In the corner on the other side of the room, a teenager stands, her fists clenched at her sides. She's screaming profanities and crying. Her makeup is so dark and smeared that the policeman standing in the open doorway isn't sure if it's heavy makeup or if she's one of those goth kids he sees downtown all the time.*

*The policeman is there because someone in the house called 911. There's a man about ten feet away from the girl, probably her father, and he's trying to calm the girl down and talk to the policeman at the same time.*

*The dispatcher said something about mental illness, and this girl sure looks crazy, the policeman says to himself. She also looks potentially dangerous—is she holding a weapon? Is she high on some street junk? Will the situation escalate?*

*In the next ten seconds, he will decide: ambulance, arrest, or takedown.*

Bipolar behaviors range from exasperating and puzzling to dangerous and terrifying. Kids with bipolar are at greater risk for drug and alcohol abuse, substances which can also aggravate their psychiatric symptoms, including rage and aggression. Their risk for suicide is higher. There's a bigger chance that they'll engage in criminal activities when they're ill and cross paths with law enforcement personnel. Many will need hospitalization during an acute crisis or severe flare-up of symptoms.

Part of managing bipolar disorder is preventing bad outcomes, but such outcomes do occur, and their impact can be felt for years. Coping with crisis takes courage, determination, and advance planning.

Your child isn't the only one at risk. Contending with the intense demands and chaos of bipolar nonstop takes its toll on everyone, especially you. An important element of bipolar management is respite for caregivers—pockets of time for you to rest and recharge. Respite may seem like a luxurious fantasy, but it is an absolute necessity. Life hygiene is just as important for you as it is for your child. If you don't take care of yourself, you'll have a hard time taking care of your child. Without proper sleep, good nutrition, and some time for the things you enjoy, you set yourself up for burnout. You're likely to become impatient, less resourceful, and less effective.

## SERIOUS AND SCARY:
## THREE MAJOR RISKS IN BIPOLAR

We call them the Big Bad Three: serious and scary outcomes that pose a significant risk for your child or teen because she has bipolar:

- Substance abuse

- Suicide

- Jail or criminal behavior

## SUBSTANCE ABUSE

*Eddie is over-the-top gleeful. He's been feeling great, so he quit taking his meds, a fact he's managed to hide from his parents. They did find a half-empty bottle of grain alcohol that he'd stashed under his bed and they are always on his case about smoking, but they don't know anything about the cocaine he's been using for the last six months or the Ecstasy he's been taking on weekends.*

From the very beginning, your child needs to hear that *he personally* has a much higher risk of both developing an addiction to drugs and alcohol and of having a bad reaction when using them. Other kids may experiment with this stuff and not suffer any ill effects, but for your child, it's like dabbling with dynamite. Drugs and alcohol may be even more seductive for him than for kids who don't have bipolar, so not only is it more dangerous for him, it may be harder for him to resist. The "high" some kids feel when they're hypomanic or manic is powerful and self-reinforcing. They want to feel more of it, which is one of the reasons they resist treatment—putting them at further risk for developing substance abuse.

Start these conversations when she's young. Make them as routine and matter-of-fact as your conversations about the importance of brushing her teeth and why she has to take medicine or go to therapy. Respect your child, even during the defiant times; she *can* learn and understand how important this is.

Help your child understand that in the short run, it can feel like drugs or alcohol "cure" her symptoms, for example, if she gets tipsy or stoned and doesn't feel so anxious at a party. But after a while, illegal drugs and alcohol make everything worse, with terrible side effects ranging from confusion and no sense of balance to death. Point out that many different chemicals are used in street drugs and there's no way to know what you're really putting into your body. She may think she's going to have a great time but end up in the hospital because the stuff she took was laced with an unknown poison.

Most kids hear about the good times these drugs are supposed to create. They don't hear the horror stories: overdoses, bad reactions, death. Make sure she realizes that getting stoned isn't all fun and games.

Ecstasy can cause life-threatening hyperthermia (very high body temperatures), which may damage the brain or other vital organs. After the initial high, GHB makes your muscles twitch and claw as in a seizure, drops your breathing, heart rate, and blood pressure to dangerously low, sometimes lethal levels, makes you vomit, takes away your gag reflex, and dumps you into coma-like consciousness. Ketamine ("special K") can cause delirium, amnesia, depression, long-term memory and cognitive deficits, and tachyarrhythmia (excessively rapid heartbeat accompanied by abnormal heart rhythm). On top of the dangers of the drugs themselves, we don't know—and neither does your child—how a particular street drug will interact with the meds your child takes for her bipolar. The combination could be lethal.

Substances we don't think of as drugs can have a big impact on kids with bipolar, too. Caffeine and nicotine alleviate distractibility and impulsivity but are so short-acting that you have to "re-dose" frequently. That leads to side effects: the jitters, difficulty sleeping, and a harder time focusing, which are the symptoms you were trying to get rid of in the first place. And of course, we know that nicotine from smoking or chewing tobacco leads to cancer and heart disease—but what kids may not know is that caffeine and nicotine can make their mood symptoms worse and may counteract some of the positive effects of their meds.

Many people believe marijuana is relatively harmless. This belief has been reinforced by recent laws that allow limited use for specific medical situations. But marijuana is not "safe and fun" for kids who have bipolar or a plus disorder. It actually contributes to their mood fluctuations and causes other symptoms that make them uncomfortable, something most kids don't realize. Smoking pot gets rid of a "nasty edge" a lot of them feel, and, for a while, it may do that better than the meds they take for bipolar. So even though their bipolar meds do a better job of stabilizing their mood and have fewer side effects, the lure of marijuana is extremely strong. Kids who get caught in this trap usually say they need marijuana to relax, calm down, or sleep. Eventually, they have to find healthier alternatives if they are going to be healthy, functioning members of society.

The central message about substance abuse you want to convey is that none of these substances work well or for long and they result in significantly worse problems, including family, legal, and behavioral problems.

Using language appropriate for your child's age and ability to understand, tell your child or teen:

1. These are toxins and your brain is still developing. A growing brain is extra susceptible to damage.

2. These substances impair your judgment. For example, alcohol makes hypersexuality worse, first because it lowers inhibitions and the teen is more likely to put herself in harm's way, and second, because it worsens her already impaired judgment, leading her to experiment with other substances or to miss the signs that she might be in a dangerous situation. It's harder to judge someone else's intentions when you're under the influence. What starts as seemingly harmless flirting at a party can disintegrate into rape or other trauma.

> Suicide is already a big risk for kids who have bipolar disorder. Alcohol and drugs increase that risk: Lowered inhibitions make it easier to act on things they might otherwise only think about.

You need to do more than talk about the dangers of substance abuse. When your child becomes an adolescent (earlier, if he's had substance abuse problems already), you need to make drug and alcohol testing part and parcel of your at-home routine. There are kits available for home use. When your teen protests that you don't trust him, don't argue. Explain that it's your responsibility as a parent to make sure he's safe and, that if problems arise, to catch them early on. You trust him to be honest, but you know that drugs do bad things to people who use them—they make honest people lie. Drug testing isn't a punishment; it's just routine, standard operating procedure.

Before prescribing medication, your clinician may require drug testing for kids who have a history of drug use or who are at risk of developing addiction. Your clinician can explain to your child that this is a safety issue, not a judgment call; we don't know what kind of reaction a street drug will have with a medication.

## SUICIDE AND THREATS OF VIOLENCE

*Six months ago, Liam took five pills from everyone's meds, beginning with his sister's Zoloft. He lined the pills up on the kitchen counter and began swallowing them quickly, one by one. His mother caught him before he made it through the entire row.*

*Liam says he wasn't feeling sad or depressed; the idea of death just came to him. His doctor talks to him about suicide and how bipolar disorder can cloud his thinking. "It sounds like you usually talk to Mom, but if she's out, could you wait?"*

*Liam's not sure, so they explore the ways he thinks about suicide and talk about how to protect him. Liam says overdosing would be his primary choice—suffocating is "too gross" and jumping out a window too painful—so staying away from meds except for the ones his mom gives him for his bipolar is a good first step.*

*The doctor emphasizes that the next time he's thinking about this, to check it out with someone else. Liam says he'll also remind himself about "good things and happy stuff." His doctor tells him that's a good idea, and that it's best to check in with Mom right away.*

*Later, Liam's mom confesses that she now locks up all prescription medications, but she hadn't realized how dangerous some over-the-counter drugs could be. She thinks about what Liam would find if he rummaged through her purse or the medicine cabinet. She routinely carries Tylenol in her purse. An overdose of Tylenol can cause severe liver damage and even death. She now locks up anything that is potentially dangerous and never carries more than four regular-strength Tylenol.*

Suicide is a significant risk for anyone who has bipolar. As many as 18% of untreated children and teens with bipolar will die from suicide. Up to 25% will attempt suicide, especially during depression. Rapid cycling—the spinning star—and substance abuse increase the risk even more. Treating bipolar decreases the risk but does not eliminate it.

It is extremely difficult to predict suicide and violent behavior. There may be warning signs, but even when you know your child is at risk and you know what to watch for, suicide, suicide attempts, and violence against others can still come as a surprise.

A lot of kids who have bipolar say they wish they were dead, threaten to kill themselves, or threaten others close to them. How do you know whether a threat means you need to sit and talk with your child or take him to the emergency room?

ALWAYS take it seriously if your child or teen talks about

or attempts suicide. It doesn't matter whether or not you believe she really intends to end her life—you need to intervene.

Psychiatric professionals try to gauge risk by looking at the *lethality* and the *risk to rescue ratio.* Attempting to overdose with pills and trying to shoot yourself are both serious suicide attempts, but overdosing is a less lethal action. Swiping and swallowing pills when Mom is in the next room has a higher chance of rescue compared to the risk of the overdose. Stockpiling pills and taking the entire stash while hiding in the woods has a lower chance of rescue and a much higher risk.

Gauging risk is useful, but it's important to know what your child was thinking and feeling. You and the clinician or therapist need to understand what led him to consider suicide. It's tough to tease out what triggered a particular episode, especially when you're not there observing or your child won't or can't explain it to you.

Keeping open lines of communication and learning to talk with your child about suicidal thoughts and feelings will help. You may not always be able to prevent a suicide attempt, but you can help your child plan for crisis situations before they happen.

Most parents are leery about talking to their kids about suicide and death. It feels worse than talking to them about the other subjects that make us uncomfortable—sex, drugs, alcohol. Yet despite that scariness and discomfort, we have to routinely address these topics.

Learn to say the words.

If she had asthma, you'd ask her if she was having trouble with wheezing or that tight feeling in her chest she gets. You'd chat with her about how to recognize an asthma attack and what to do.

She has bipolar; you ask if she's been feeling depressed or thinking about death or suicide lately. You chat with her routinely about what she should do if she does start thinking about them. Who would she talk to? If she can't talk to you, whether because she doesn't want to or because you're not available, who else could she talk to? Push her to think this through: Perhaps it's another relative, her therapist, a twenty-four-hour hotline, or a trusted friend.

A teen in mid-rage who's holding the knife he just grabbed from the kitchen counter while screaming that he wants to kill himself is scarier than a teen in mid-rage who's slamming doors and knocking the kitchen chairs over while screaming the same thing. In both cases, the top priority is de-escalation and everyone's safety. After the dust settles, help him examine what triggered the outburst, including what he's feeling and whether he was serious about injuring himself or ending his life. You may discover that the threats stemmed from the heat of the moment: He had no plan, had not been thinking about suicide at all, and said things he didn't mean; the biggest danger was that he'd continue to escalate. If you have the slightest doubt that he's telling the truth, contact your clinician or therapist for advice.

If he admits that he's feeling suicidal, take him to the nearest emergency room for an evaluation. Do not wait: Most people threaten suicide or talk about it before they make an actual attempt. (See "Suicide Warning Signs," below.)

Some kids will threaten parents or siblings when they're angry. These threats need to be examined with the same care as suicide threats. Are there other elements that indicate danger? Is there a reason for the threats?

*When Daryl got mad at his little sister (which happened frequently), he threatened to stab her. His therapist questioned him about these threats, and Daryl admitted that he made them so his sister would quit bugging him. He wasn't and isn't going to stab her, but he does need to find a better way to interact with his sister that doesn't involve scaring her away.*

*In therapy and at home, he's practicing other things to say when he wants her to leave him alone, and he's working toward not threatening* at all. His therapist is helping him understand the broader impact of his words. For example, if his sister tells her teacher that Daryl wants to stab her, the teacher may call the Department of Social Services, which may decide that for safety's sake Daryl or his sister should live with foster families instead of with their parents.

Daryl's threats to his sister result primarily from his impulsivity, immaturity, and poor social skills. He has a clear and accurate understanding of what triggers his outbursts, though he isn't always able to use his new skills to prevent them. His moods are fairly stable, he shows no other signs that hint at violent or self-destructive behavior, and he's beginning to use more appropriate ways to handle disagreements with his sister.

Colin's situation is much different. He's a ninth-grader at a therapeutic boarding school. Yesterday, he erupted in a rage so severe that the school insisted that he be evaluated before being allowed to return. They want to know if it's safe—for Colin and for others at the school— for him to return to class.

During his evaluation, Colin slouches low in his chair. His voice, when he finally answers the doctor's question about what happened at school, is low and tight with anger. He doesn't make eye contact. He begins listing the people he was angry with and others who made him angry. He's still furious with his fifth-period teacher. He wants to go back to school but not to that teacher or class.

His doctor asks Colin if at any time, he wanted to hurt the teacher or anyone else. Was he out of touch with reality during this episode? Colin says no to both questions and admits that he is still angry. He says it's the teacher's fault, that this teacher singles him out, and the school always takes the teacher's side. Colin's mother tries to explain what the teacher might be thinking, which only makes Colin more irritated.

The doctor continues to press Colin for details that will help clarify the core issue: Is Colin a threat to others or himself? He doesn't have plans to hurt anyone; he doesn't have access to weapons; and the school, which targets kids with problems like Colin's, has excellent safety and security measures in place. Colin's illness has always included a *lot of paranoia, but it seems focused on one particular class today, not the whole world. His mood might be less stable, but it's hard to tell if that's bipolar and paranoia getting worse, a reaction to the school situation, or due to something else they haven't identified yet.*

*They finally decide that Colin can return to school but he will either be excused from the fifth-period class or a guidance counselor or other neutral third party will sit with him in the class. The doctor also makes a slight adjustment to Colin's meds to gain better control over his anger and paranoia.*

*Colin's mom and the doctor are still worried, but this is the best decision they can make given the information they have.*

*Colin didn't make it to fifth period the next day; he lost it halfway through first period. He attacked a teacher and had to be physically restrained. He was transported to the hospital emergency room and from there to inpatient psychiatric treatment. Both the doctor and Colin's mom wondered if there was something they missed. Did Colin's day begin as smoothly as his mom thought? Did she underestimate the potential for danger because she's gotten used to his being angry? Did his doctor miss other clues during his evaluation?*

Knowing that a child's risk for violent behavior is high is not the same thing as being able to predict if and when he will be violent or suicidal. No matter how skilled and attentive parents, teachers, and clinicians are, predicting violent or suicidal behavior is difficult. Kids with bipolar do sometimes lose control, but most kids most of the time are not a danger to others or themselves.

We don't want to accuse a child of being a threat when he isn't. We also want to err on the side of safety for everyone.

SUICIDE PREVENTION LIFELINE

If you or someone you care about is in crisis and you need help right away, call the National Suicide Prevention Lifeline:

**1-800-273-TALK**
**1-800-273-8255**

They're available twenty-four hours a day, seven days a week. All calls are confidential.

*Para obtener asistencia en español:* 1-888-628-9454

TTY: 1-800-799-4TTY (1-800-799-4889)

Profile on myspace.com:
www.myspace.com/suicidepreventionlifeline

More info about the National Suicide Prevention Lifeline: www.suicidepreventionlifeline.org

## Suicide Warning Signs

You may believe that your child or teen won't consider suicide, that he "doesn't have it in him." Unfortunately, bipolar can cloud your child's thinking; he might have it in him because he has bipolar. It's better to err on the side of caution. It's extremely difficult to predict suicide attempts, but the following factors increase the risk.

*Plan?* Has your child talked about methods or formulated a plan? Has he been surfing websites about suicide or talking to others online about methods?

*Access?* Does your child have access to weapons, drugs (including prescription and over-the-counter medications), or environments where he could easily be in harm's way?

*Prior Attempts?* Trying once increases the chances that he'll try again.

*Risk to Rescue Ratio?* How risky is the method she tried compared to the chances for rescue?

*Drugs or Alcohol?* Lowered inhibitions increase the risk of acting on things she might otherwise only think about.

*Peer Acceptance or Encouragement?* Does she have friends who accept or romanticize questionable behavior? This type of peer support can intentionally or inadvertently encourage suicide. (See "Pros and Cons of Peer Pressure," below.)

*In the News?* Celebrity suicides as well as the suicide of people he knows (classmates, other peers, adults in the community) raise the risk for him, too.

*Family History?* Family history of attempted or completed suicide, mental disorders, or substance abuse increases your child's risk.

*Unstable Mood?* Bipolar disorder can cloud your child's thinking and reasoning abilities.

*Cutting and Burning?* Cutting and burning are self-destructive behaviors generally associated with depression. They're not suicidal behaviors per se, but they are a sign of severe emotional stress and as such should be taken seriously. Most kids who cut are not trying to kill themselves, but they are in so much emotional pain, they cut or burn as a way to distract themselves from the emotional pain and to release tension and anxiety.

## JAIL: CRIMINAL BEHAVIOR, CONDUCT DISORDER, AND BIPOLAR

*Until he was thirteen, Jake was cheerful and helpful, with a delightful sense of humor. His first manic episode hit just before seventh grade. He began lying, vandalizing property, shoplifting, and bullying other kids. He was a swaggering braggart and a show-off. He showed no remorse for his actions and boasted that he'd never be caught. It took three years to find a combination of meds to stabilize Jake's moods—but when they stabilized, his conduct disorder disappeared. He's now an ethical young adult with a strong conscience.*

The symptoms of bipolar disorder can cross the line from "difficult to deal with" to dangerous, illegal, or both. Criminal behavior driven by mental illness is still criminal behavior, and the consequences become more severe as your child gets older. Mania-fueled rage, meltdowns, and destructive behavior can be misconstrued by police and other authority figures, leading to potentially disastrous outcomes.

Nobody is "born bad," but some children do seem wired for trouble from the beginning. In others, mild oppositional and conduct disorders surface gradually, occasionally, or not at all. And for some, conduct disorder appears full blown, seemingly out of nowhere.

It isn't always obvious whether the behaviors we call "oppositional defiance" (ODD) and "conduct disorder" (CD) are distinct conditions, separate from each other and bipolar. It is clear that both ODD and CD are common bipolar-plus disorders, and that mania fuels both of them. When CD appears out of the blue or its symptoms suddenly escalate, it's almost always in conjunction with bipolar disorder.

There is no known treatment for conduct disorder or "criminality," but we can treat the rage, aggression, impulsivity, and poor judgment that drive much of criminal behavior. In other words, we treat the mood disorder, and the conduct disorder problems improve, too.

Kids with bipolar and conduct disorder need closer supervision than those with bipolar alone. Treating the mania dampens the CD fire, but there is still a greater risk for criminal behavior. You want to do everything you can to prevent that and to keep your child or teen out of the juvenile justice system.

If your kid is a thrill seeker (and especially if he gravitates toward illegal activities), get him involved in legitimate activities that generate the adrenaline charge he needs—extreme sports, emergency room medicine, search and rescue teams, and law enforcement.

If your teen breaks the law, he may have to take the consequences that society doles out, even though the behavior was
caused by his illness. In rare cases, and with appropriate
placement, this can be an important wake-up call that con-
vinces him that he needs to stick with his treatment. More
likely, it will reinforce his belief that he's a criminal, which can
become a self-fulfilling prophecy. His medical care, including
psychiatric care, may be beyond your control when he's in the
juvenile detention center or jail. Changes in medication, including disputes over diagnosis resulting in no treatment at
all, lead to worse symptoms, more trouble, and reinforcement
of his "I'm a bad guy" identity.

If you think you can't prevent your child from doing these
kinds of behaviors, consider enrolling her in a residential
setting—a therapeutic boarding school or other around-the-
clock program—where her treatment can be tightly controlled while she develops the skills and maturity she needs
for the "real world."

### Working with Police and Other First Responders

*Fourteen-year-old Loren tells the story calmly. "I was angry," he says,
"but I wasn't going to do anything. I was just holding the knife,
squeezing it really hard. I got angrier and squeezed harder, that's all.
Mom finally took it away from me, but I wasn't going to do anything,
honest." Later, Loren's mom confesses that she thought about calling
the police. Loren's taller than she is now, and she worries about
whether she can keep her other children safe when Loren's mood goes
haywire. She worries about protecting him from himself, too; he's cut
himself before, and he's gone through periods when he was obsessed
with weapons. But she's even more worried about calling the police,
who might not understand what's really going on.*

Bipolar disorder, like other "invisible" disabilities, causes behaviors that are easy to misinterpret. The standard procedures followed by police and other law enforcement personnel

assume they're dealing with a standard brain generating standard body language, behavior, and reactions.

Two basic scenarios are likely to involve the police: They call you, or you call them.

Mania fuels your teen's aggression, impulsivity, and grandiosity; he does something stupid, illegal, or both and gets caught. To the police, he's arrogant, defiant, obnoxious, and says he doesn't care that what he's done is wrong. When they confront him, his behavior gets worse, not better. The police contact you to tell you he's been arrested.

Your teen's in the midst of a horrible rage storm. Nothing you do to help her de-escalate is working. You call 911 because things have reached the point where you cannot ensure everyone's safety by yourself, or because you need help restraining her and getting her to the emergency room or psychiatric hospital, or because you hope the "uniform" will break through some of the grandiosity and denial. When the police arrive, your teen, who is in a severe state of agitation and has practically no insight into what's happening, escalates even more. To the police, the situation looks like domestic violence, the outcome of horrible parenting, or a criminal who needs to be taken out of commission as quickly as possible.

In both scenarios, the way the police respond may not be the ideal approach for handling the situation.

So: What can you as a parent do to work best with law enforcement? How can you improve safety for all concerned, get the assistance your family needs, and minimize the potential for miscues?

Be proactive.

You need to disclose that your child has bipolar disorder. You can and should convey this information during the crisis (when you're talking to the 911 operator, for example), but you should also reach out to your local law enforcement and emergency services before you need them.

*Ask your local 911 emergency call center to include and "red flag" your child's information in their database.* When a call comes in to 911 from your address, the flagged information will come up on the operator's screen, and the operator can alert the first responders (police, paramedics) *before* they arrive.

Some 911 call centers have systems in place to flag information. Massachusetts uses a "Disability Indicator Form" that includes a "cognitive impairment" category.* The standardized form doesn't allow for details, but when a call comes in, a special code alerts the operator that someone at that address may require special assistance during an emergency. (Note that if you call from a different address, the code doesn't automatically appear, because it's tied to your physical home address.)

Other emergency call centers may be able to include more detailed information, and a few may be unable or unwilling to include any. If the call center turns down your request, keep asking, alone or in combination with your support group, advocacy groups, and other organizations whose members would benefit from having specific information incorporated into the emergency database.

*Ask your local law enforcement agency (police department, sheriff's office) and fire and rescue departments to include information about your child in their database now,* so it will be readily available if it's ever needed. Not all agencies can, but it's worth asking.

*Ask if personnel receive training about pediatric bipolar disorder and other mental illnesses.* Meet with the chief of police, sheriff, shift commanders, and other supervisors to discuss the issues, individually or in partnership with other groups. Push for training that embraces the "special tactics" you use with your child every day.

If they say no, keep asking. Be persistent; you're making a reasonable request that benefits everyone. The more field

---

*www.mass.gov/Eeops/docs/setb/disability_form.pdf and www.mass.gov/Eeops/docs/ setb/disability_info.pdf, accessed May 7, 2007.

officers and first responders know about the situation they're encountering, the better they'll be able to respond appropriately and effectively.

*Create an "emergency information handout."* Keep copies of it taped to the refrigerator, near the phone, in your car, in your purse or wallet—in short, anywhere you may need the information quickly and anywhere it can be found easily if you're not available. Not all emergencies are caused by bipolar. If you're knocked unconscious in a car accident, the emergency information handout will give paramedics crucial information about your child. You can give copies of the handout to the law enforcement and emergency service agencies—it has the information you want flagged in the databases—and to anyone else you deem appropriate, including neighbors, teachers, or relatives.

The purpose of the handout is to help others know what to do in case of crisis or emergency, whether or not you're available. It should include:

- Your child's full name

- A current photo and physical description (height, weight, eye and hair color, any scars or identifying marks)

- Names, phone numbers (home, work, cell, pager), and addresses of parents, other caregivers, and emergency contact persons

- Name and phone numbers (including after-hours number or pager) for the psychiatrist, advanced practice nurse, or other medical professional who prescribes your child's medications

- Your child's diagnosis including plus disorders

- A list of all medications, including the dosages and when they're taken

- Any other medical, dietary, or sensory issues

- Brief descriptions of likes, dislikes, and behaviors that are probably not what they seem, for example, "direct confrontation and asserting authority causes agitation and aggressive behavior to escalate; may be unable to follow verbal directions or commands"

- Brief descriptions of techniques you use to help your child, for example, "appear to retreat; lower voice tone"

- Blueprint or map of your home

Remember to update the form when meds or other information change.*

### Hypersexuality and Allegations of Abuse

Preschoolers are fascinated with bodies. That's developmentally normal and easy to deal with for most parents and teachers.

Not so with older children and teens. Teachers and other adults often believe that any inappropriate sexual talk or behavior is caused by sexual abuse, and, as required by law, report their suspicions to the Department of Social Services (DSS) or Child Protective Services (CPS).

Teachers, neighbors, or other caring adults might also contact DSS/CPS if they think your child shows signs of physical or emotional abuse. For example, if your child's behavior is self-destructive (cutting, burning) or aggressive (punching

*Thanks to Dennis Debbaudt, Autism Risk & Safety Management.

walls, smashing windows), an observer might assume that the scars, bruises, and lacerations were from abuse.

DSS/CPS is required by law to investigate everything that is reported to them. It's their job.

You can make their job easier and protect yourself from false or misguided accusations by documenting your child's behavior and its causes. Your documentation should include the emergency information handout (see "Working with Police and Other First Responders," above) as well as a record of aggressive, self-injurious, hypersexual, or other extreme behavioral episodes; the names of anyone who witnessed them; and anything you did to help alleviate the situation. This documentation could be a copy of your tracking chart or journal or a separate document you create for your "just in case" file. If you can, include photographs of bruises or injuries with an explanation of what happened and the date.

This documentation helps DSS/CPS understand that your child's behavior stems from her mood disorder and that you are pursuing appropriate treatment. The investigators will be able to wrap up their report quickly and accurately.

### Pros and Cons of Peer Pressure
Kids with bipolar disorder usually don't fit in with the standard "popular" crowd. They often end up in a peer group with kids who tolerate or fuel inappropriate behavior. The problem with these groups isn't necessarily peer pressure, but the lack of it. The "bad peers" aren't pressuring your child to do drugs or engage in other risky behavior, but they accept the behavior, and they don't pressure your child *not* to do drugs or engage in risky behavior.

Your child hears friends talk about how much fun they had on Ecstasy or how much relief they felt by cutting and are seduced more than coerced into trying the behavior. The same dynamic can increase the risk of any dangerous or illegal behavior, including suicide. If your daughter tells her friends she's been thinking about suicide and their response is acceptance (ranging from "Sure, okay" to "Wow, that would be so cool"), it can reinforce her belief that she should try it. She and a friend might form a suicide pact or promise to keep a suicide plan secret. Even if the friend is worried or afraid, she might believe that betraying your daughter's trust is worse than telling someone about the plan.

Kids with bipolar struggle with their illness every day. They may have already survived trauma, drug abuse, and suicide attempts. They've probably been rejected by friends and been the subject of gossip when their symptoms flared; lost friends because their ability to be a friend changed when they were ill; and been separated from friends because of hospitalization, separate classrooms, or special schools. Their lives and life experiences are so different from those of "regular" kids that the regular kids have a hard time connecting with them.

Every child, bipolar or not, needs a peer group, a place where they're accepted. Some kids find others who have similar difficulties or who understand brain disorders or who are simply more accepting of differences. Sharing stories, having inside jokes, and identifying with other members of the group are all part of bonding and becoming part of the group. The group helps its members assimilate the hard knocks of life and provides a buffer against the rejection of other groups.

There will be times when you'll have to draw the line and say not this group, not this friend, a task which gets more difficult as she passes through her teen years. Equally important is to accept and welcome her friends whenever possible. Form solid relationships with them, and you'll be a trusted source of support when times get tough. Her friends will be more willing to come to you with their concerns, and you'll be more tuned in to what's going on within the group. The better you know the group and its members, the better you'll be able to guide your child through the pros and cons of her peer group.

## HOSPITALIZATION

*Initially, meds decreased twelve-year-old Anna's irritability and moodiness, but within a week, her depression became so severe she needed to be hospitalized. When her parents told her they were taking her to the hospital, she said okay. When they got there, she got mad at them because they wouldn't take her home. Anna says at first, the hospital was scary. She didn't know anyone and didn't know what to expect. She remembers watching the kids who had attempted suicide and thinking that since she hadn't tried that, the other kids were obviously a lot sicker than she was—so why was she here? She felt nothing would help, which was another reason why they should let her go home.*

*Her family came in for visits and meetings. Anna attended daily group meetings with other patients but felt too anxious and shy to participate. After a few days, she felt safe, more comfortable around the other kids and in group meetings, and began to participate a little. Anna's doctor also changed her meds and adjusted the dosage during this time. After a week in the hospital, her moods were stable enough that she could go home.*

You might think of hospitalization as a last resort for dire emergencies, but for most children and teens with bipolar, it's simply part of long-term treatment. Hospitals aren't magic, but at the right time and for the right reasons, hospital care is useful and appropriate.

Because so many children and teens with bipolar need to be hospitalized at some time, investigate your options now, before you need them. You don't want to be arguing with your insurance carrier over coverage or frantically trying to decide which hospital or emergency room to go to when you're in the midst of a crisis.

Call your insurance carrier to get the details about coverage. You need to know how many days are covered, whether you need to use a specific hospital, and authorization or admission procedures. These procedures include who to call during business hours, after hours, or over the weekend and whether you can call after your child has already been admitted.

One of the most common questions insurance companies will ask before authorizing a hospital stay is, "Is your child a danger to himself or others?"

The very question can send you into retreat. Things are bad, but are they that bad?

Remember that you grow accustomed to challenging and extreme behavior because you deal with it every day. You've decided your child needs hospitalization, a decision you never take lightly, a decision you've made because your child's illness *is* that bad. When you call your insurance provider to request authorization to hospitalize your child, the answer to this question is *YES*.

Not all hospital emergency rooms have psychiatric care. Ask your doctor for recommendations, and verify that the options are covered by your insurance.

Acute Psychiatric Services (APS), whether available through a hospital's emergency room or as an independent service, are usually your first choice, but you may end up waiting a long time, twenty hours or more, before they can admit your child. In this case, it may make more sense to go to your local emergency room, if they can admit your child promptly. Since you won't know which choice is the best until you need the emergency care, be prepared for both.

### Reasons to Take Your Child to the Hospital

- She's a danger to herself or others, and you can't keep her or those around her safe. This includes immediate danger such as suicide threats or attempts or violent and out-of-control behavior (for example, kicking out the windshield, attacking and injuring a sibling) as well as sustained behavior which hasn't been helped by other interventions such as adjusting dosage or timing her medication.

- He's ingested something suspicious. You can't know how much he took or what it might have been combined with. Remember that many things we don't think are dangerous, aspirin or Tylenol, for example, can be life-threatening.

- Symptoms are extremely severe; you need to disrupt the cycle and make meds changes faster than can be safely done as an outpatient.

- You need to confirm a diagnosis or document the severity of the illness; more hospitalizations indicate a more severe illness.

### What to Expect

Hospitalization can be frightening for both you and your child. It might be the first time you've been separated overnight. It's hard to leave your child, to feel she's safe and protected, when it seems like the other patients are in worse shape or much older or younger than your child.

It's hard for your child, too. Even if she's agreed to go and wants the help available there, don't be surprised if she changes her mind and wants to go home immediately.

Hospitals, like juvenile detention centers and jails, are scary for another reason: Your child may be with kids who have done some scary things. You aren't just worried about your child's safety; you're worried she'll learn behaviors she wouldn't have thought of if she never met these kids.

But meeting tough and scary kids in these settings may be the reality check your child needs. For some kids, this experience is a wake-up call about consequences—they're "scared straight." Others realize they aren't as unique or bad off as they thought they were. If the reality check connects, they'll often be more responsible about their own treatment because they finally recognize what could happen if they don't take their treatment seriously.

Admission to the hospital usually includes a meeting with you, your child, and one or more people from the hospital's psychiatric team. In most places, you'll be ushered out quickly after the meeting, which can make you feel even more anxious. A few programs are following the lead of their medical counterparts and allowing parents to stay at the hospital with their child. A hospital staff person will search your child's belongings for anything that is potentially dangerous—belts, sharp objects such as jewelry, tweezers, pocket knives, and nail clippers, any liquids that might be toxic if swallowed—and either lock up the items for safekeeping or give them to you to take home.

The next day, you'll meet with the hospital team—social worker, psychiatric floor staff, and others—and may also meet one-on-one with other specialists who are involved with your child's care. If your child was admitted during the weekend, you'll probably see the clinician who is covering admissions that weekend, then meet the rest of the team the following Monday.

### Goals for Hospitalization

*Ethan was admitted to the hospital after attacking and injuring his brother, the final straw of increasingly severe problems and mood instability. Ethan's mother had heard about a forty-five-day emotional needs summer camp and suspected it would be a good placement for him. She and his advanced nurse practitioner pushed the hospital team to do an evaluation to determine the suitability of the camp for Ethan.*

*Ethan was already an identified special needs student with an IEP. Since the camp was the least restrictive environment—he'd already tried everything else the school offered, and ongoing hospitalization was more restrictive than he needed—the school paid for the cost of the camp. The camp staff continued the close meds supervision as well as providing other support services.*

*With the combination of hospital intervention, meds changes, and a new plan including the emotional needs camp, Ethan left the hospital in much better shape than when he'd arrived, stable enough that he could benefit from the camp program.*

Most health insurance policies don't cover extensive stays, so if you have particular goals, you need to move them along quickly. In a sense, you need to be your child's case manager and advocate.

For example, one of the most common goals is to change medication to achieve better mood stability. You can facilitate this simply by providing the contact information for your child's outpatient clinician (the person who regularly pre-scribes your child's medication) to the hospital psychiatrist working with your child. And it's easy to do—give the hospital clinician a copy of your emergency information handout. If you haven't already done so, fax a signed information release form to your clinician along with the name, phone and fax numbers, and e-mail address of the hospital clinician.

Through the hospital setting, you can identify and pursue additional services your child needs and get help to put them rapidly in place. These can include

- fast-tracking eligibility for Department of Mental Health services;

- specifying a school placement and creating a plan for the school your child is returning to (for example, regular school with proper supports, or a recommendation for a therapeutic day or residential school);

- new therapy, including emotional support, anger management, in-home services and specialists, and one-on-one support;

- parent support services, including crisis management training and respite services;

- case management services to help you access therapeutic services your child needs;

- addressing drug and alcohol problems, including arranging for detoxification, rehabilitation, and drug resistance programs;

- making certain evaluations higher priority—an evaluation for a specific program or a comprehensive exam, such as a neuropsychological evaluation;

- lab work to monitor drug levels or other conditions;

- addressing medical issues that may be contributing to your child's difficulties, for example, seeing an endocrinologist for diabetes or a pediatric neurologist for suspected problems.

The hospital isn't a cure-all; roughly half of the families say hospitalization helped, and half say their child was the same or worse at the end of their stay. Occasionally, parents report that their child learned new "bad behaviors" from the other hospitalized kids. Sometimes, the improvement you see in the hospital turns out to be just a breather before your ill child comes home and the next round of struggles begins.

Which brings us to an often-overlooked goal to consider: How are your other kids doing while their sibling is in the hospital?

Siblings often feel resentful, under siege, fearful, or forgotten. How do your children feel and behave when the pressure and chaos of bipolar are out of the way? This can be a good opportunity to listen to the concerns your children have and to brainstorm together on ideas for what to do in the future. You may discover that you need to make some adjustments in "family management"—finding ways for your children to experience life, at least some of the time, without the stress of bipolar after your ill child returns home.

## RESPITE FOR PARENTS

Parents often sacrifice personal life and private time trying to meet the demands of raising kids who have bipolar. There are nonstop physical demands on your time—handling the latest crisis, advocating for school services, juggling finances, and more. There are nonstop emotional demands—the pain of watching your child struggle, the worry about how that child's illness will affect your other kids, the disagreements with your spouse over what to do and how to do it, the frustration, anger, resentment—and love—that drive you to find the best ways to help your child.

You need a break.

A few minutes every day for yourself, to recharge and de-stress. A longer stretch of time when you can manage it. Time alone, time with your spouse or friends.

Respite helps protect you—from exhaustion, burnout, even depression and stress-related illnesses. It is healthy and appropriate to take some time for yourself. Here are some ways other parents have fit respite time into their lives.

There's no easy way for Eric and Sandra to get away. Two of their three children have bipolar, and Sandra herself developed adult-onset bipolar a year after her younger daughter was diagnosed. Her respite routine includes daily walk-and-talks with a friend and, several times a week, a hot bath, complete with aromatic oils and candles. She and her husband also share "afternoon tea" almost every day. She admits it sounds a little silly, but she finds this late afternoon pause very calming.

\* \* \*

Maria drops her kids at school—all three have bipolar, each with a different cluster of plus disorders—and heads to the pool. This particular pool is part of a facility that was founded specifically for people with developmental delays and other cognitive disabilities and their families. She qualifies because one of her sons has Asperger's syndrome as well as bipolar. She swims laps and socializes a little with other caregivers. She's missed several months recently because she was home-schooling one of her boys while her IEP appeal wound its way through the system. Now that he's back in school, she's back swimming laps for a half hour every morning.

Kristen hoped to spend a week honeymooning with her new husband. Plenty of friends and relatives volunteered to let her son, David, stay with them. There were no takers at all for his big sister, Amy, and no money to hire a live-in specialist. Because Amy's illness was so severe, Kristen was finally able to get respite services through her state's Department of Mental Health.

During their twice-a-year family visits, Michael's grandparents did "trial runs" caring for him and his siblings, making sure they could handle everything from meds and meltdowns to the parenting strategies Michael's parents used. In addition to providing respite for Michael's parents during these visits, they were well prepared to care for their grandchildren, in-cluding Michael, when his parents took a longed-for and much-delayed two-week vacation.

In her search for respite, Melinda Suits founded an agency. The number-one request from families in Melinda's parent support group was for respite. "We need a break—it's so intense. And regular babysitters don't work," she says.

Melinda, mom to a young son with bipolar and the facilitator of the Fort Collins chapter of EMPOWER Colorado, joined forces with Liz Terrell-Phillips, therapist and board member of the Federation of Families of Northern Colorado, to form a new respite agency, DREAM (Day by day Respite, Education, and Advocacy for Mental health, www.idreamof respite.org). They began offering respite services in 2006 and are now a United Way agency.

Their original plan called for a physical facility similar to the respite programs offered for people with physical disabilities, but they quickly realized that their program could be both more flexible and more cost effective if they used a different approach. DREAM trains respite care providers, who then work as independent consultants for families. DREAM also has a family intake specialist who helps identify the type of care a family needs, a respite coordinator who keeps in touch with families, a program director, and a development (fundraising) director. They're governed by a volunteer board of directors made up of parents, therapists, advocates, and philanthropists.

Depending on the needs of the family, the care provider may stay with the child at the family's home or take the child on field trips and to community programs or events. Families and care providers establish goals to work toward during respite care, too, for example, the care provider might work with a child on social or anger issues.

Crisis management and respite care are opposite sides of the caregiver coin. Tackling the latest crisis is infinitely more difficult if you're exhausted, stressed out, and perpetually overwhelmed. Take the time to restore yourself—you and your child will both be healthier for it.

# Bibliography

American Psychiatric Association. *Diagnostic and Statistical Manual of Mental Disorders: DSM-IV.* Washington, DC: American Psychiatric Association, 1994.

Biederman, Joseph, Janet Wozniak, Kathleen Kiely, J. Stuart Ablon, Stephen Faraone, Eric Mick, Elizabeth B. Mundy, and Ilana Kraus. "CBCL Clinical Scales Discriminate Prepubertal Children with Structured Interview-Derived Diagnosis of Mania from Those with ADHD." *Journal of the American Academy of Child & Adolescent Psychiatry* 34, no. 4 (April 1995): 464–471.

Biederman, Joseph, M. A. McDonnell, Janet Wozniak, T. Spencer, M. Aleardi, R. Falzone, and Eric Mick. "Aripiprazole in the Treatment of Pediatric Bipolar Disorder: A Systematic Chart Review." *CNS Spectrums* 10, no. 2 (February 2005): 141–148.

Biederman, Joseph, Stephen V. Faraone, Eric Mick, Janet Wozniak, L. Chen, C. Ouellette, A. Marrs, P. Moore, J. Garcia, Douglas Mennin, and E. Lelon. "Attention-Deficit Hyperactivity Disorder and Juvenile Mania: An Overlooked Comorbidity?" *Journal of the American Academy of Child & Adolescent Psychiatry* 35, no. 8 (1996): 997–1008.

Carlson, G. A., and D. P. Cantwell. "Unmasking Masked

Depression in Children and Adolescents." *The American Journal of Psychiatry* 137, no. 4 (1980): 445–449.

Carlson, G. A., and F. K. Goodwin. "The Stages of Mania: A Longitudinal Analysis of the Manic Episode." *Archives of General Psychiatry* 28, no. 2 (1973): 221–228.

Debbaudt, Dennis. "Plan Your Response to an Autism Emergency." *Dennis Debbaudt's Autism Risk & Safety Newsletter,* Winter 2007. http://www.autismriskmanagement.com/Winter2007 .html#PYR (accessed July 19, 2007).

___. Dennis Debbaudt's Autism Risk and Safety Management website. http://www.autismriskmanagement.com (accessed July 19, 2007).

Dimeff, Linda, and Marsha M. Linehan. "Dialectical Behavior Therapy in a Nutshell." *The California Psychologist* 34 (2001): 10–13. http://www.dbtselfhelp.com/DBTinaNutshell.pdf (accessed July 18, 2007).

Doyle, Alysa E., Timothy E. Wilens, Anne Kwon, Larry J. Seidman, Stephen V. Faraone, Ronna Fried, Allison Swezey, Lindsey Snyder, and Joseph Biederman. "Neuropsychological Functioning in Youth with Bipolar Disorder." *Biological Psychiatry* 58, no. 7 (2005): 540–548.

Frank, Ellen, D. J. Kupfer, M. E. Thase, A. G. Mallinger, H. A. Swartz, A. M. Fagiolini, V. Grochocinski, P. Houck, J. Scott, W. Thompson, and T. Monk. "Two-Year Outcomes for Interpersonal and Social Rhythm Therapy in Individuals with Bipolar I Disorder." *Archives of General Psychiatry* 62, no. 9 (2005): 996–1004.

Fristad, Mary A., and Jill S. Goldberg-Arnold. *Raising a Moody Child: How to Cope with Depression and Bipolar Disorder.* New York: Guilford Press, 2004.

Giedd, Jay. "Child and Adolescent Psychiatry: New Views from Brain Imaging." Summary of speaker presentation at National Institute of Mental Health Alliance for Research Progress Science Meeting, January 24, 2005, Bethesda, MD. Page 5. http://www.nimh.nih.gov/health/outreach/alliance/alliancereport 24jan05.pdf (accessed July 19, 2007).

Greene, Ross W. *The Explosive Child: A New Approach for Understanding and Parenting Easily Frustrated, Chronically Inflexible Children.* New York: Harper, 2005.

Klein, D. C., Robert Y. Moore, and Steven M. Reppert. *Suprachiasmatic Nucleus: The Mind's Clock.* New York: Oxford University Press, 1991.

Kowatch, R. A., Mary A. Fristad, B. Birmaher, K. D. Wagner, R. L. Findling, and M. Hellander. "Treatment Guidelines for Children and Adolescents with Bipolar Disorder: Child Psychiatric Workgroup on Bipolar Disorder." *Journal of the American Academy of Child & Adolescent Psychiatry* 44, no. 3 (March 2005): 213–235.

Leibenluft, Ellen. "Circadian Rhythms Factor in Rapid-Cycling Bipolar Disorder." *Psychiatric Times* 23, no. 5 (May 1996): http://www.psychiatrictimes.com/p960533.html (accessed July 18, 2007).

Leibenluft, Ellen, Eric A. H. Turner, Susana Feldman-Naim, Paul J. Schwartz, Thomas A. Wehr, and Norman E. Rosenthal. 1995. "Light Therapy in Patients with Rapid Cycling Bipolar Disorder: Preliminary Results." *Psychopharmacology Bulletin* 31, no. 4 (1995): 705–710.

Ma, Lybi. "Interview: The Fisher Queen." *Psychology Today,* November/December 2001. http://psychologytoday.com/articles/pto-20011101-000022.html (accessed July 19, 2007).

Manji, Husseini. "Anxiety and Depression Research: New Ideas from the NIMH MAP." Summary of speaker presentation at National Institute of Mental Health Alliance for Research Progress Science Meeting, January 24, 2005, Bethesda, MD. Page 3. http://www.nimh.nih.gov/health/outreach/alliance/alliancereport24jan05.pdf (accessed November 20, 2007).

McClellan, J., and J. Werry. "Practice Parameter for the Assessment and Treatment of Children and Adolescents with Bipolar Disorder." *Journal of the American Academy of Child & Adolescent Psychiatry* 46, no. 1 (2007): 107–125. http://www

.aacap.org/galleries/PracticeParameters/JAACAP_Bipolar_2007 .pdf (accessed July 18, 2007).

Moore, Constance M., Joseph Biederman, Janet Wozniak, Eric Mick, M. Aleardi, M. Wardrop, M. Dougherty, T. Harpold, P. Hammerness, E. Randall, and P. F. Renshaw. "Differences in Brain Chemistry in Children and Adolescents with Attention Deficit Hyperactivity Disorder with and without Comorbid Bipolar Disorder: A Proton Magnetic Resonance Spectroscopy Study." *The American Journal of Psychiatry* 163, no. 2 (February 2006): 316–318.

National Institute of Mental Health (U.S.). *Breaking Ground, Breaking Through: The Strategic Plan for Mood Disorders Research of the National Institute of Mental Health.* NIH publication no. 03-5121. Bethesda, MD: U.S. Dept. of Health and Human Services, National Institutes of Health, 2003. http://www .nimh.nih.gov/strategic/mooddisorders.pdf (accessed July 18, 2007).

———. "Child and Adolescent Bipolar Disorder: An Update from the National Institute of Mental Health." NIH publication no. 00-4778. Bethesda, MD: U.S. Department of Health and Human Services, Public Health Service, National Institutes of Health, 2000. http://www.nimh.nih.gov/publicat/bipolar update.cfm (accessed July 18, 2007).

———. "Fear Circuit Flares as Bipolar Youth Misread Faces." National Institute of Mental Health (NIMH) press release, May 30, 2006. http:www.nimh.nih.gov/press/bipolarfaces .cfm (accessed July 19, 2007).

———. Report, National Institute of Mental Health Alliance for Research Progress Science Meeting, January 24, 2005, Bethesda, MD. http://www.nimh.nih.gov/health/outreach/ alliance/alliancereport24jan05.pdf (accessed July 19, 2007).

Pavuluri, Mani N., Patricia A. Graczyk, David B. Henry, Julie A. Carbray, Jodi Heidenreich, and David J. Miklowitz. "Child- and Family-Focused Cognitive-Behavioral Therapy for Pediatric Bipolar Disorder: Development and Preliminary Results."

*Journal of the American Academy of Child & Adolescent Psychiatry* 43, no. 5 (2004): 528.

Pavuluri, Mani N., Lindsay S. Schenkel, Subhash Aryal, Erin M. Harral, S. Kristian Hill, Ellen S. Herbener, and John A. Sweeney. "Neurocognitive Function in Unmedicated Manic and Medicated Euthymic Pediatric Bipolar Patients." *The American Journal of Psychiatry* 163, no. 2 (February 2006): 286–293.

REBT Network. Web site devoted to the work of Albert Ellis and Rational Emotive Behavior Therapy. http://www.rebtnetwork .org/index.html (accessed July 19, 2007).

Rich, Brendan A., Deborah T. Vinton, Roxann Roberson-Nay, Rebecca E. Hommer, Lisa H. Berghorst, Erin B. McClure, Stephen J. Fromm, Daniel S. Pine, and Ellen Leibenluft. "Limbic Hyperactivation During Processing of Neural Facial Expressions in Children with Bipolar Disorder." *Proceedings of the National Academy of Sciences of the United States of America* 103, no. 23 (2006): 8900–8905. http://www.pnas.org/cgi/content/ abstract/0603246103v1 (accessed July 18, 2007).

Simpson, G. A., B. Bloom, R. A. Cohen, S. Blumberg, and K. H. Bourdon. 2005. "U.S. Children with Emotional and Behavioral Difficulties: Data from the 2001, 2002, and 2003 National Health Interview Surveys." *Advance Data* no. 360 (2005): 1–13.

Soares, J. C., and J. J. Mann. "The Anatomy of Mood Disorders— Review of Structural Neuroimaging Studies." *Biological Psychiatry* 41, no. 1 (1997): 86–106.

———. "The Functional Neuroanatomy of Mood Disorders." *Journal of Psychiatric Research* 31, no. 4 (1997): 393–432.

Tillman, R., B. Geller, K. Bolhofner, J. L. Craney, M. Williams, and B. Zimerman. "Ages of Onset and Rates of Syndromal and Subsyndromal Comorbid DSM-IV Diagnoses in a Prepubertal and Early Adolescent Bipolar Disorder Phenotype." *Journal of the American Academy of Child & Adolescent Psychiatry* 42, no. 12 (December 2003): 1486–1493.

Wozniak, Janet. "Recognizing and Managing Bipolar Disorder in

Children." *The Journal of Clinical Psychiatry* 66, suppl. 1 (2005): 18–23.

Wozniak, Janet, Joseph Biederman, Stephen V. Faraone, Heather Blier, and Michael C. Monuteaux. "Heterogeneity of Childhood Conduct Disorder: Further Evidence of a Subtype of Conduct Disorder Linked to Bipolar Disorder." *Journal of Affective Disorders* 64, no. 2 (2001): 121–131.

Wozniak, Janet, Joseph Biederman, Kathleen Kiely, J. Stuart Ablon, Stephen V. Faraone, Elizabeth Mundy, and Douglas Mennin. "Mania-Like Symptoms Suggestive of Childhood-Onset Bipolar Disorder in Clinically Referred Children." *Journal of the American Academy of Child & Adolescent Psychiatry* 34, no. 7 (1995): 867–876.

*Appendix A*

## SUMMARY OF THE DSM-IV DIAGNOSTIC CRITERIA FOR BIPOLAR DISORDER

### Criteria for Manic Episode

A. A distinct period of abnormally and persistently elevated, expansive, or irritable mood, lasting at least 1 week (or any duration if hospitalization is necessary).

B. During the period of mood disturbance, three (or more) of the following symptoms have persisted (four if the mood is only irritable) and have been present to a significant degree:

(1) inflated self-esteem or grandiosity

(2) decreased need for sleep (e.g., feels rested after only 3 hours of sleep)

(3) more talkative than usual or pressure to keep talking

(4) flight of ideas or subjective experience that thoughts are racing

(5) distractibility (i.e., attention too easily drawn to unimportant or irrelevant external stimuli)

(6) increase in goal-directed activity (either socially, at work or school, or sexually) or psychomotor agitation

(7) excessive involvement in pleasurable activities that have a high potential for painful consequences (e.g., engaging in unrestrained buying sprees, sexual indiscretions, or foolish business investments)

C. The symptoms do not meet criteria for a Mixed Episode.

D. The mood disturbance is sufficiently severe to cause marked impairment in occupational functioning or in usual social activities or relationships with others, or to necessitate hospitalization to prevent harm to self or others, or there are psychotic features.

E. The symptoms are not due to the direct physiological effects of a substance (e.g., a drug of abuse, a medication, or other treatment), or a general medical condition (e.g., hyperthyroidism).
   **Note:** Manic-like episodes that are clearly caused by somatic antidepressant treatment (e.g., medication, electroconvulsive therapy, light therapy) should not count toward a diagnosis of Bipolar I Disorder.

### Criteria for Major Depressive Episode

A. Five (or more) of the following symptoms have been present during the same 2-week period and represent a change from previous functioning; at least one of the symptoms is either (1) depressed mood or (2) loss of interest or pleasure.
   **Note:** Do not include symptoms that are clearly due to a general medical condition, or mood-incongruent delusions or hallucinations.

   (1) depressed mood most of the day, nearly every day, as indicated by either subjective report (e.g., feels sad or empty), or observation made by others (e.g., appears tearful). Note: In children and adolescents, can be irritable mood.

   (2) markedly diminished interest or pleasure in all, or almost all, activities most of the day, nearly every day (as indicated by either subjective account or observation made by others)

   (3) significant weight loss when not dieting or weight gain (e.g., a change of more than 5% of body weight in a month), or decrease or increase in appetite nearly every day. Note: In children, consider failure to make expected weight gains.

(4) insomnia or hypersomnia nearly every day
(5) psychomotor agitation or retardation nearly every day
    (observable by others, not merely subjective feelings of
    restlessness or being slowed down)
(6) fatigue or loss of energy nearly every day
(7) feelings of worthlessness or excessive or inappropriate
    guilt (which may be delusional) nearly every day (not
    merely self-reproach or guilt about being sick)
(8) diminished ability to think or concentrate, or indecisive-
    ness, nearly every day (either by subjective account or as
    observed by others)
(9) recurrent thoughts of death (not just fear of dying), re-
    current suicidal ideation without a specific plan, or a
    suicide attempt or a specific plan for committing suicide.

B. The symptoms do not meet criteria for a Mixed Episode.

C. The symptoms cause clinically significant distress or impairment in social, occupational, or other important areas of functioning.

D. The symptoms are not due to the direct physiological effects of
a substance (e.g., a drug of abuse, a medication) or a general
medical condition (e.g., hypothyroidism).

E. The symptoms are not better accounted for by bereavement;
i.e., after the loss of a loved one, the symptoms persist for longer
than 2 months, or are characterized by marked functional impairment, morbid preoccupation with worthlessness, suicidal
ideation, psychotic symptoms, or psychomotor retardation.

## Criteria for Mixed Episode

A. The criteria are met both for a Manic Episode and for a Major
Depressive Episode (except for duration) nearly every day during at least a 1-week period.

B. The mood disturbance is sufficiently severe to cause marked
impairment in occupational functioning or in usual social activities or relationships with others, or to necessitate hospitalization

to prevent harm to self or others, or there are psychotic features.

C. The symptoms are not due to the direct physiological effects of a substance (e.g., a drug of abuse, a medication, or other treatment) or a general medical condition (e.g., hyperthyroidism).

> **Note:** Mixed-like episodes that are clearly caused by somatic antidepressant treatment (e.g., medication, electroconvulsive therapy, light therapy) should not count toward a diagnosis of Bipolar I Disorder.

Reprinted with permission from the *Diagnostic and Statistical Manual of Mental Disorders, Fourth Edition, Text Revision,* (Copyright © 2000 by American Psychiatric Association).

*Appendix B*

## ADHD SYMPTOM CHECKLIST

The formal description of ADHD includes "distractible," "impulsive," and "inattentive"—but what do those look like? This checklist provides examples of behaviors that might be signs of ADHD. You can use this list to describe or track your child's behavior, or simply use it as a way to think about the symptoms that worry you or interfere with your child's ability to function. NOTE: Remember that even if your child has many of the symptoms listed here, it doesn't necessarily mean he has ADHD (or only ADHD). Your clinician must rule out other possible causes (including mood disorders) before making a diagnosis.

## ADHD SYMPTOM CHECKLIST

**Difficulty remaining seated**
Leaves seat in classroom or other setting in which sitting is expected

**Fidgety**
Fidgets with items, hands, feet; squirms in chair

**Difficulty playing quietly**
Hard time engaging in quiet activities that aren't stimulating or that don't involve a lot of activity (leisure activities, doing fun things quietly)

**Talks excessively**
Talks more than most people

**Shifts activities**
Jumps from one activity to another without finishing the first activity

**Difficulty sustaining attention**
Hard time paying attention during tasks or fun activities (NOT including stimulating activities, e.g., computer, TV, video games)

**Difficulty following instructions**
Isn't able to follow through on detailed instructions, instructions with multiple steps, and/or doesn't finish work

**Easily distracted**
Almost anything—a noise, someone whispering in the back of the room, someone else fidgeting, etc.—can distract from the task at hand

**Interrupts or intrudes**
Interrupts conversations or intrudes on situations (seems rude, oblivious, or impulsive)

**Blurts out answers**
Answers before hearing the whole question, finishes others' sentences for them

**Difficulty waiting for his/her turn**
Can't wait! Difficulty waiting; impatience; inability to stand in line

**Acts before thinking**
Gets in trouble for saying or doing things or rushing into
things without considering the consequences or results

**Loses things**
Loses or misplaces important things (keys, files, papers, homework, coat, shoes, etc.)

**Doesn't listen**
Unable to listen when spoken to directly—not an oppositional,
"I won't listen," but more a reflective, daydreaming, or difficulty in paying attention throughout the entire conversation

**Doesn't pay close attention to detail**
Makes careless mistakes in work or on tests, misses important
details

**Disorganized**
Papers or notebook are a mess, difficulty organizing a task or
activity, can't find things (not because they're actually lost
but because things are so disorganized that there's no
good way to find them)

**Avoidance or extreme dislike of mental tasks**
Avoids, dislikes, is reluctant to engage in work that requires
sustained mental effort (e.g., detail-oriented homework or
tasks that are boring)

**Often forgetful**
Misses appointments; forgets books, papers, homework; needs
lots of reminders to keep track of activities or tasks

**Hyperactive: often "on the go" or "driven by a motor"**
Actual physical activity

**Hyperactive: feels restless**
Feels restless or an uncomfortable sense of needing to be doing something all or most of the time

*Appendix C*

# SYMPTOMS OF PEDIATRIC MANIA
## FROM THE MGH PEDIATRIC MANIA
## SYMPTOM CHECKLIST

The following list of mood and behavior symptoms is from the MGH Pediatric Mania Symptom Checklist used by researchers and clinicians at Massachusetts General Hospital. You can use the list to describe or track your child's behavior, or simply use it as a way to think about the symptoms that worry you or interfere with your child's ability to function. NOTE: Remember that even if your child has many of the symptoms listed here, it doesn't necessarily mean she has bipolar disorder (or only bipolar disorder). Your clinician must rule out other possible causes for the symptoms, examine the intensity, severity, and types of symptoms, and carefully consider other factors before making a diagnosis.

For additional charts, descriptions, and ideas for keeping track of symptoms, see the checklists and other information available from S.T.E.P. Up for Kids, Inc., http://www.stepup4 kids.com.

**Mood State: Euphoria**
Felt or acted excessively good, high, excited, or hyper in a way
that was not appropriate for his/her age
Had excessive or inappropriate laughing fits
Had silly, goofy, or giddy moods in a way that was not appro-
priate for his/her age or acted babyish or immature

**Mood State: Irritability**
Was extremely irritable, angry, cranky, grouchy, hostile, or un-
cooperative
Experienced explosive anger
Was assaultive, destructive, or threatening

**Increased Activity/Agitation**
Did a lot with friends or at school, in a frenzied or pressured
way
Took on big projects, such as starting a business, rearranging
furniture, or other projects that seemed large in scope for
him/her
Was restless or highly energetic as compared to peers or self
Had excessive focus on one activity or topic to an extreme or
odd degree

**Hypersexuality**
Had age-inappropriate sexual thoughts or actions
Was preoccupied with bathroom humor, rude remarks involv-
ing body parts or sexual matters
Touched self or others inappropriately
Exposed body inappropriately
Involved others in sexual play in a way that posed a problem

**Decreased Need for Sleep**
Needed fewer hours of sleep per night, as compared to peers
or self
Can function on less sleep than others his/her age
Did not feel tired even when sleeping less

**Talkativeness (code as less severe if only during rage)**
Talked a lot, loudly or fast as compared to peers or self
Could not stop talking, or difficult to interrupt

**Flight of Ideas/Racing Thoughts**
Was unable to stop jumping between thoughts
Had difficulty keeping track of thoughts or changed topics a
    lot
Complained of racing thoughts or that his/her brain was too
    active

**Distractibility**
Had trouble concentrating as compared to peers or self
Was significantly bothered by minor distractions as compared
    to peers or self

**Psychosis**
Seemed to be hearing or seeing things
Acted paranoid, as if everyone were against him/her
Acted grandiose to a degree that was bizarre or out of touch
    with reality
Had bizarre behaviors that were out of touch with reality

**Grandiosity**
Felt or acted overly self-confident or overestimated own ability
    to do things in actions or bragging
Felt stronger, smarter, or more powerful than most people or
    acted as if this were so, as if he/she could do anything
Flagrant disregard for household or school rules, as if he/she
    were above the rules
Was especially bossy/controlling

**Activities Showing Poor Judgment**
Did impulsive or reckless things that caused trouble or made
    bad decisions causing trouble
Felt especially lucky, took chances, or acted like a daredevil

Spent money excessively or wanted to buy a lot
Was disinhibited in seeking out people or strangers

**Appearance**
Needed reminder about cleanliness or appeared disheveled
Had odd ideas about how to appear
Dressed in odd or sexually provocative manner in makeup,
    jewelry, or clothing
Dressed inappropriately for weather or situation

**Insight**
Denied that he/she has problem
Refused help or treatment because doesn't need it
Did not take responsibility for actions or blamed others inap-
    propriately

*Appendix D*

MEDICATIONS

## MOOD STABILIZERS: LITHIUM

| Generic Name | Common Brand Names | Side Effects, Notes |
|---|---|---|
| Lithium | Eskalith, Lithium, Lithotabs, Lithium citrate, Eskalith CR, Lithobid | Can have negative effect on kidney and thyroid functioning, thus blood tests at least twice per year are essential to monitor safety. Works best at a certain blood level and can be dangerous at high levels. |

## MOOD STABILIZERS: ANTICONVULSANTS

| Generic Name | Common Brand Names | Side Effects, Notes |
|---|---|---|
| Valproate | Depakote | Works best at a certain blood level; blood tests also monitor liver functioning. Can have harmful effects on liver and pancreas functioning. Can be sedating. |
| Carbamazepine | Tegretol, Carbatrol, Equetro | Works best at a certain blood level; can be dangerous at high levels. Blood tests also measure white blood cell count, which, especially early in treatment, needs close monitoring to check for the possibility of a dangerous decrease. Allergic skin rash can be dangerous. |
| Oxcarbazepine | Trileptal | Related chemically to carbamazepine but with fewer side effects. Low sodium a risk, but blood tests generally not required. |

## MOOD STABILIZERS: ANTICONVULSANTS

| Generic Name | Common Brand Names | Side Effects, Notes |
|---|---|---|
| Lamotrigine | Lamictal | FDA has placed a warning for youths under age sixteen due to risk of severe allergic skin rash (Stevens-Johnson syndrome), which can occur in any age group. Skin rash less likely with very slow upward dose taper. Dose must be adjusted if used with Depakote, which can increase the Lamictal level. No blood tests required, but levels can be tested. |
| Topiramate | Topamax | Cognitive clouding is the major side-effect concern. Decrease in appetite means this medication is often used in combination to avoid weight gain from other medications. |

## MOOD STABILIZERS:
## ATYPICAL OR NOVEL ANTIPSYCHOTICS

| Generic Name | Common Brand Names | Side Effects, Notes |
|---|---|---|
| Risperidone | Risperdal | Prolactin elevation, sedation, muscle spasm and movement side effects, tardive dyskinesia, weight gain, diabetes, and lipid elevations |
| Olanzapine | Zyprexa, Zydis | Sedation, muscle spasm and movement side effects, tardive dyskinesia, weight gain, diabetes, and lipid elevations |
| Quetiapine | Seroquel | Sedation, muscle spasm and movement side effects, tardive dyskinesia, weight gain, diabetes, and lipid elevations |

## MOOD STABILIZERS:
## ATYPICAL OR NOVEL ANTIPSYCHOTICS

| Generic Name | Common Brand Names | Side Effects, Notes |
|---|---|---|
| Ziprasidone | Geodon | Sedation, muscle spasm and movement side effects, tardive dyskinesia, weight gain, diabetes, and lipid elevations; cardiac effect with prolongation of the QTc interval (slower heart rate, which may increase the risk of a heart arrhythmia) |
| Aripiprazole | Abilify | Sedation, muscle spasm and movement side effects, tardive dyskinesia, diabetes, and lipid elevations |
| Clozapine | Clozaril | Sedation, muscle spasm and movement side effects, tardive dyskinesia, weight gain, diabetes, and lipid elevations; can cause a life-threatening decrease in white blood cell count, so requires weekly or biweekly blood tests for safety monitoring |

## OTHERS

| Generic Name | Common Brand Names | Side Effects, Notes |
|---|---|---|
| Gabapentin | Neurontin | Generally safe medication; sedation is the main side effect |
| Clonazepam | Klonopin | Generally safe medication; sedation is the main side effect; can be cognitively clouding; low risk of addiction |
| Lorazepam | Ativan | Generally safe medication; sedation is the main side effect; can be cognitively clouding; low risk of addiction |
| Antidepressants | | Major concern is that these medications can exacerbate manic symptoms in those with bipolar illness. Various antidepressants have specific side effects including sexual dysfunction, sedation, weight gain, and worsening of depression. |

## OTHERS

| Generic Name | Common Brand Names | Side Effects, Notes |
|---|---|---|
| Conventional antipsychotics | Haldol, Thorazine, Mellaril, and Trilafon | Sedation, weight gain, tardive dyskinesia (occurs in high rates with long-term use); some of these medications require cardiac monitoring |
| Omega-3 fatty acids | OmegaBrite Coromega Nordic Naturals (and other brands) | Fishy taste, upset stomach |

*Appendix E*

# RESOURCES: WEB SITES, SUPPORT GROUPS, AND ADVOCACY ASSISTANCE

## American Academy of Child & Adolescent Psychiatry (AACAP)

www.aacap.org

AACAP is a nonprofit professional medical association dedicated to treating and improving the quality of life for children, adolescents, and families affected by mental, behavioral, or developmental disorders. Its members actively research, evaluate, diagnose, and treat psychiatric disorders, and the AACAP distributes information through its Web site and elsewhere in an effort to promote an understanding of mental illnesses and remove the stigma associated with them, advance efforts in prevention of mental illnesses, and assure proper treatment and access to services for children and adolescents.

*See also:* Bipolar practice parameters: www.aacap.org/galleries/PracticeParameters/JAACAP_Bipolar_2007.pdf

## American Foundation for Suicide Prevention

www.afsp.org

The American Foundation for Suicide Prevention (AFSP) is a nonprofit organization dedicated to understanding and preventing suicide through research and education, and to reaching out to people with mood disorders and those affected by suicide.

## Bazelon Center for Mental Health Law
www.bazelon.org
The Judge David L. Bazelon Center for Mental Health Law (previously called the Mental Health Law Project) is a legal advocate for people with mental disabilities. The center's mission is to protect and advance the rights of adults and children who have mental disabilities. The center envisions an America where people who have mental illnesses or developmental disabilities exercise their own life choices and have access to the resources that enable them to participate fully in their communities.

## *bp Magazine* and *bp Canada*
www.bphope.com/ and www.bphope.ca
*bp Magazine* and its Canadian counterpart *bp Canada* are online magazines for those living with bipolar disorder (children and adults) and a community for people with shared concerns and varied experiences. Each issue features helpful health tips and information about bipolar and conveys the personal stories of challenge and success that each person who lives with bipolar disorder faces. *bp Magazine*'s goal is to promote hope and harmony for bipolar individuals and the ones who love them.

## Child & Adolescent Bipolar Foundation (CABF)
www.bpkids.org
CABF is a parent-led, nonprofit, Web-based membership organization of families raising children diagnosed with, or at risk for, pediatric bipolar disorder.

## Children and Adults with Attention Deficit/ Hyperactivity Disorder (CHADD)
www.chadd.org
*See also:* National Resource Center on AD/HD (NRC)
CHADD is a membership-based nonprofit organization for people with ADHD and their families. CHADD has over sixteen thousand members in two hundred local chapters throughout the U.S. Chapters offer support for individuals, parents,

teachers, professionals, and others. In addition to local chapters, CHADD produces *Attention!* magazine (for members) and sponsors an annual conference.

**Dennis Debbaudt's Autism Risk & Safety Management**
www.autismriskmanagement.com
In 1994 Dennis Debbaudt's book *Avoiding Unfortunate Situations* became the first to address the interactions between law enforcement professionals and people with autism. Since then he has become known as the world's leading authority on the development of curriculum training tools and techniques for law enforcement professionals. His recommendations also apply to many children and teens with other brain disorders, including bipolar disorder.

**Depression and Bipolar Support Alliance (DBSA)**
www.dbsalliance.org and ndmda.org
DBSA is a nonprofit patient-directed national organization that fosters an environment of understanding about the impact and management of depression and bipolar disorder by providing up-to-date, scientifically based tools and information written in language the general public can understand. DBSA also supports research to promote more timely diagnosis, develop more effective and tolerable treatments, and discover a cure, and it works to ensure that people living with mood disorders are treated equitably.

**EMPOWER Colorado**
www.empowercolorado.com
EMPOWER Colorado is a family-run organization offering support, education, and advocacy to families with children and youth who have social, emotional, or mental health challenges. The organization has formally partnered with other organizations, each with a unique focus and expertise. By working together through these partnerships, they are better able to help families with their many different needs as well as reduce the number of outside referrals.

## Healthy & Ready to Work (HRTW)

www.hrtw.org/healthcare
Maternal and Child Health Bureau's Division of Services for Children with Special Health Care Needs (MCHB/DSCSHN) (www.mchb.hrsa.gov) has funded the development and demonstration of model Healthy & Ready to Work (HRTW) state programs focused on children and youth with special healthcare needs (CYSHCN). The Web site includes information to help caregivers and young people understand their health needs, be involved in their healthcare decision-making, and transition from child-centered to adult-oriented systems of care.

## I.D.E.A.S.

www.ideasnpo.org
I.D.E.A.S. (Individual Development to Education, Attitudes, & Solutions Corporation) advocates for children with disabilities, advises and informs the parents of children with disabilities, and provides training to enable parents and others to better advocate for children who have special needs, so that they may secure the appropriate educational services and supports for these children.

## Independent Educational Consultants Association (IECA)

www.iecaonline.com
The Independent Educational Consultants Association (IECA) is a nonprofit, international professional association representing full-time, experienced, independent educational advisors. IECA member consultants counsel students and their families in the selection of educational programs, based on the student's individual needs and talents.

## International Society for Bipolar Disorders

www.isbd.org/portal

A forum of researchers, clinicians, advocacy groups, and individuals to foster ongoing international collaboration, education, research, and advances in all aspects of bipolar disorders, including treatment. ISBD also publishes the journal *Bipolar Disorders—An International Journal of Psychiatry and Neurosciences*.

## Juvenile Bipolar Research Foundation

www.jbrf.org

The Juvenile Bipolar Research Foundation is a charitable organization dedicated to the support of research for the study of early-onset bipolar disorder. In addition, JBRF sponsors an online educational forum for parents, educators, and other professionals, intended to establish and encourage an ongoing national dialogue that will promote a better understanding of the educational challenges that confront children with juvenile-onset bipolar disorder.

## The Legal Center for People with Disabilities and Older People

www.thelegalcenter.org

The Legal Center is an independent public interest nonprofit specializing in civil rights and discrimination issues. The center protects the human, civil, and legal rights of people with mental and physical disabilities, people with HIV, and older people throughout Colorado.

## MADI Resource Center

www.mgh.harvard.edu/madiresourcecenter

www.moodandanxiety.org

*See also:* Schoolpsychiatry.org

The mission of the Mood & Anxiety Disorders Institute (MADI) Resource Center is to educate patients, families, caregivers, and the community about mood and anxiety disorders in order to increase understanding, instill hope, facilitate recovery, and improve lives. The center offers information, resources, and support through its Web sites, reading materials, support groups, and seminars for the public.

### National Alliance on Mental Illness (NAMI)

www.nami.org
NAMI is the largest grassroots mental health organization in the United States dedicated to improving the lives of people living with serious mental illness, and their families. There are NAMI organizations in every state and in over eleven hundred local communities across the country who join together to meet the NAMI mission through advocacy, research, support, and education. NAMI is dedicated to the eradication of mental illnesses and to the improvement of the quality of life of all whose lives are affected by these diseases.

### National Institute of Mental Health

www.nimh.nih.gov/publicat/index.cfm
www.nimh.nih.gov/healthinformation/index.cfm
NIMH is the leading United States federal agency for research on mental and behavioral disorders. Its mission is to reduce the burden of mental illness and behavioral disorders through research on the mind, brain, and behavior. The Web site includes many articles (including understandable summaries) about mood disorders and lists of resources, ongoing research studies, and other information about bipolar disorder.

### National Resource Center on AD/HD (NRC)

www.help4adhd.org
*See also:* Children and Adults with Attention Deficit/Hyperactivity Disorder (CHADD)
The National Resource Center on AD/HD (NRC), a program of CHADD, is the nation's clearinghouse for science-based information about all aspects of attention deficit/hyperactivity disorder (ADHD). The NRC was created to provide information about ADHD to professionals and the general public.

## National Suicide Prevention Lifeline

1-800-273-TALK (1-800-273-8255)

www.suicidepreventionlifeline.org

The National Suicide Prevention Lifeline is a twenty-four-hour, toll-free suicide prevention service available to anyone in suicidal crisis. Its mission is to provide immediate assistance to anyone seeking mental health services. *If you need help, please dial* **1-800-273-TALK (8255)** and they will route your call to the closest crisis center. Call for yourself or someone you care about. Your call is free and confidential.

## Parent/Professional Advocacy League

www.ppal.net/default

The Parent/Professional Advocacy League (PAL) is an organization of more than four thousand Massachusetts families and professionals who advocate on behalf of children with emotional, behavioral, and mental health needs and their families. PAL advocates for supports, treatments, and policies that enable families to live in their communities in an environment of stability and respect. PAL provides support, training, and technical assistance to a large network of PAL family support specialists who in turn provide support, information, and advocacy resources to thousands of families across Massachusetts.

## Partnership for Workplace Mental Health

www.workplacementalhealth.org

The Partnership for Workplace Mental Health advances effective employer approaches to mental health by combining the knowledge and experience of the American Psychiatric Association and employer partners. The partnership delivers educational materials; provides a forum to explore mental health issues and share innovative solutions; and promotes the business case for quality mental health care, including early recognition, access to care, and effective treatment.

**Schoolpsychiatry.org**
www.massgeneral.org/schoolpsychiatry
www.schoolpsychiatry.org
*See also:* MADI Resource Center
Schoolpsychiatry.org is a joint project of the School Psychiatry Program and the Mood & Anxiety Disorders Institute (MADI) Resource Center, both of the Department of Psychiatry at Massachusetts General Hospital (MGH). The schoolpsychiatry.org Web site was created for parents, educators, clinicians, and clinicians-in-training to identify and support the needs of children and adolescents with mental health conditions. This site contains information about recognizing and treating a range of mental health disorders in young people and making appropriate accommodations at school and at home.

**Screening for Mental Health (SMH)**
www.mentalhealthscreening.org
Screening for Mental Health, Inc., (SMH) is a nonprofit organization that first introduced the concept of large-scale mental health screenings with its flagship program National Depression Screening Day in 1991. SMH programs now include both in-person and online programs for depression, bipolar disorder, generalized anxiety disorder, post-traumatic stress disorder, eating disorders, alcohol problems, and suicide prevention.

**S.T.E.P. Up for Kids**
www.stepup4kids.com
S.T.E.P. Up for Kids, Inc., is a nonprofit organization established to assist parents; families; legal, medical, and mental health professionals; teachers; school administrators; teens; and children by providing the necessary education, support, and tools that will create a better understanding of and a more enriching life for children and adolescents afflicted with pediatric-onset bipolar disorder and other behavioral and emotional disorders.

## BOOKS FOR CHILDREN, INCLUDING THOSE WHO HAVE BIPOLAR DISORDER

*Brandon and the Bipolar Bear: A Story for Children with Bipolar Disorder,* by Tracy Anglada, Trafford Publishing, 2004.

*My Bipolar Roller Coaster Feelings Book and Workbook* and *Answer Mountain* by Bryna Hebert, Trafford Publishing, 2005.

*The Storm in My Brain: Kids and Mood Disorders,* by the Child & Adolescent Bipolar Foundation and the Depression and Bipolar Support Alliance, 2003.

*Turbo Max: A Story for Siblings of Bipolar Disorder,* by Tracy Anglada, bpchildren.com, 2002.

*When Nothing Matters Anymore (Revised & Updated Edition): A Survival Guide for Depressed Teens,* by Bev Cobain, Free Spirit Publishing, 2007.

## MORE INFORMATION AND RESOURCES FOR SCHOOL SUPPORT SERVICES, SPECIAL EDUCATION, AND IEPS

*Your state's department of education.* If you're not sure what your state's educational agency is called or how to contact them, ask at the school or the public library. The state educational agency (which is not the same as your school district) is responsible for ensuring that all children who have disabilities receive a free appropriate public education in their state.

*Advocacy groups and agencies.* Check with local support groups, the state department of education, and your child's doctor or therapist for recommendations.

### Books and CDs

*The Everyday Guide to Special Education Law: A Handbook for Parents, Teachers, and Other Professionals,* by Randy Chapman, Esq. 2005, The Legal Center for People with Disabilities and Older People, Denver, Colorado.

*Guía de la Ley de Educación Especial—Una Guía para Padres, Maestros y Otros Profesionales Académicos,* by Randy Chapman, Esq. and Heinrich Hispanidad, The Legal Center for People with Disabilities and Older People, Denver, Colorado, 2007. (Spanish translation of *The Everyday Guide to Special Education Law;* both the Spanish and English text are included on every page.)

*The Complete IEP Guide: How to Advocate for Your Special Ed Child,* by Lawrence M. Siegel, Nolo Press, 2007.

*Straight Talk About Psychological Testing for Kids,* by Ellen B. Braaten and Gretchen Felopulos, the Guilford Press, 2003.

*Individual Education Plans: Involved Effective Parents,* by Alison B. Seyler and Barbara E. Buswell, PEAK Parent Center, Inc., Colorado Springs, Colorado, 2001.

*The ABCs of Educational Advocacy* and *What Is Pediatric Bipolar Disorder: A Resource for Educators,* interactive CDs available from the Child and Adolescent Bipolar Foundation, www.bpkids.org.

**Web sites with information about attorney and special education legal issues**

*American Bar Association Consumers' Guide to Legal Help* (www.abanet.org/legalservices/findlegalhelp/home.cfm) provides lists of legal resources by state in the United States.

*Council of Parent Attorneys and Advocates, Inc.* (COPAA) (www .copaa.org) was established to be a national voice for special education rights, to promote excellence in advocacy, and to secure high-quality educational services for children with disabilities by ensuring the availability and quality of legal and advocacy resources for parents of children with all types of disabilities.

*LawHelp* (www.lawhelp.org) helps low- and moderate-income people find free legal aid programs in their communities and answers to questions about their legal rights.

*The Legal Center for People with Disabilities and Older People* (www.thelegalcenter.org), a nonprofit agency specializing in civil rights and discrimination issues, protects the human, civil and legal rights of people with mental and physical disabilities, people with HIV, and older people throughout Colorado.

*Special Education Law Blog* (http://specialedlaw.blogs.com) is a special education legal resource discussing case law, news, practical advocacy advice, and developments in state and federal laws, statutes, and regulations. Postings include insight and sometimes humor from Charles P. Fox, a Chicago, Illinois, attorney who is also the parent of a child with special needs, and other guest authors.

*Wrightslaw* (www.wrightslaw.com) is a Web site with extensive and detailed information about special education law, education law, and advocacy for children with disabilities. Wrightslaw also produces publications and training programs.

**Web sites with good information about research-based methods, curriculum-based assessments, learning disabilities, and advocacy**

*All Kinds of Minds* (www.allkindsofminds.org) helps students who struggle with learning measurably improve their success in school and life by providing programs that integrate educational, scientific, and clinical expertise.

*International Center for the Enhancement of Learning Potential* (ICELP) (www.icelp.org) was established to continue and expand the educational and psychological work initiated by Professor Reuven Feuerstein, based on the theories of Structural Cognitive Modifiability and Mediated Learning Experience, which serve as a basis for three applied systems: the Learning Potential Assessment Device (LPAD), Instrumental Enrichment (IE) cognitive intervention program, and Shaping Modifying Environment. The licensed distributor and the lead authorized training center for Feuerstein programs in North America is *iRi* (www.iriinc.us).

*LD Online* (www.ldonline.org) seeks to help children and adults reach their full potential by providing accurate and up-to-date information and advice about learning disabilities and ADHD.

*Lindamood-Bell* (www.lindamoodbell.com) is an organization dedicated to enhancing human learning, founded in 1986 by Nanci Bell, Patricia Lindamood, and Phyllis Lindamood, the authors of critically acclaimed programs that teach children and adults to read, spell, comprehend, and express language.

*National Center for Learning Disabilities* (www.ncld.org) provides essential information about learning disabilities, early literacy and learning resources, support for adolescents and adults with learning disabilities, public policy, and advocacy tools.

*Schoolpsychiatry.org* (www.massgeneral.org/schoolpsychiatry), a joint project of the School Psychiatry Program and the Mood & Anxiety Disorders Institute (MADI) Resource Center, both of the Department of Psychiatry at Massachusetts General Hospital (MGH), is committed to enhancing the education and mental health of every student in every school.

*SchwabLearning.org* (www.schwablearning.org) is dedicated to providing reliable, parent-friendly information about learning disabilities from experts and parents.

*STARFISH Advocacy Association* (SAA) (www.starfishadvocacy.org) creates opportunities for joy through learning and sharing information, resources, and support within the community for children with neurological disorders and their families.

*U.S. Department of Education* (www.ed.gov) was formed to promote student achievement and preparation for global competitiveness by fostering educational excellence and ensuring equal access. Among other tasks, the agency is charged with prohibiting discrimination and ensuring equal access to education.

## About the Authors

JANET WOZNIAK, MD, the director of pediatric bipolar research at Massachusetts General Hospital, is assistant professor of psychiatry there as well as at Harvard Medical School.

MARY ANN MCDONNELL, APRN, BC, is the executive director of S.T.E.P. Up for Kids, Inc., a nonprofit organization supporting children and teens with bipolar disorder. A clinical university instructor, she also maintains a private practice in pediatric psychopharmacology.

JUDY FORT BRENNEMAN is an award-winning writer, owner of Greenfire Creative, LLC, and a long-time advocate for kids with hidden disabilities.

# Index